Praise for NO SECRETS, NO LIES

"A compelling collection of stories and survival strategies."
—*Essence*

"One of the most important books some of us will ever read."
—Mary Mitchell, *Chicago Sun-Times*

"[Robin D.] Stone's understanding of, and empathy for, incredibly painful situations comes through on every page, and her techniques for beginning to deal with them are compassionate and straightforward."
—*Publishers Weekly*

"A comprehensive look at perhaps the most underreported of all crimes."
—Rubén Rosario, *Saint Paul Pioneer Press*

"Stone's new book breaks the silence about sexual assault within black families."
—*Detroit Free Press*

"Robin is doing a healer's work."
—Katti Gray, *Newsday*

"Powerful stories . . ."
—*Library Journal*

"*No Secrets, No Lies* opens the door to understanding and healing."
—*Today's Black Woman*

"Powerful, positive, and right on time, Robin Stone's *No Secrets, No Lies* demystifies sexual abuse in the Black community and empowers survivors. A must-read for anyone who cares about the health of their family and of children everywhere."
—Faira Chideya, author of *The Color of Our Future* and *Don't Believe the Hype*

P9-DBY-740

"In *No Secrets, No Lies* Robin D. Stone provides invaluable insights and tools for both families and mental health professionals to address the ever-present problem of sexual abuse that has been hidden too long."

—Kim Singleton, Ed.D., clinical psychologist and author of
Broken Silence

"*No Secrets, No Lies* presents an empowering and healing approach to childhood sexual abuse from a culturally relevant perspective. It provides insight into dysfunctional family dynamics and abuse patterns from the view of victims and perpetrators. Without pathologizing victimization, Robin D. Stone systematically fosters the development of ego strength and survival strategies. Every psychologist and therapist should use *No Secrets, No Lies* as an invaluable guide and resource with clients who have experienced sexual trauma."

—Darlene Powell-Garlington, Ph.D., clinical psychologist
and coauthor of *Different and Wonderful: Raising Black
Children in a Race-Conscious Society*

NO SECRETS, NO LIES

How Black Families Can Heal

from Sexual Abuse

ROBIN D. STONE

HARLEM MOON
BROADWAY BOOKS
New York

Published by Harlem Moon, an imprint of Broadway Books, a division of Random House, Inc.

A hardcover edition of this book was originally published in 2004 by Broadway Books, a division of Random House, Inc.

NO SECRETS, NO LIES. Copyright © 2004 by Robin D. Stone. All rights reserved. No part of this book may be reproduced or transmitted in any form or by any means, electronic or mechanical, including photocopying, recording, or by any information storage and retrieval system, without written permission from the publisher. For information, address Broadway Books, a division of Random House, Inc.

PRINTED IN THE UNITED STATES OF AMERICA

HARLEM MOON, BROADWAY BOOKS, and the HARLEM MOON logo, depicting a moon and a woman, are trademarks of Random House, Inc. The figure in the Harlem Moon logo is inspired by a graphic design by Aaron Douglas (1899–1979).

Visit our website at www.harlemmoon.com

First Harlem Moon trade paperback edition published 2004

Book design by Erin L. Matherne and Tina Thompson

The Library of Congress has cataloged the hardcover edition as follows:
Stone, Robin D.
   No secrets, no lies : how black families can heal from sexual abuse / Robin D. Stone.—1st ed.
      p. cm.
   Includes bibliographical references.
   1. Sexually abused children—Family relationships. 2. African American families. 3. Incest victims—Family relationships. I. Title.
HQ71.S767 2004
362.883'089'96073—dc22   2003065385

ISBN 978-0-7679-1345-4

To my family, and for all our families

"As we share with others, we offer them the power of our healing experiences."

Byllye Avery, health activist and founder,
National Black Women's Health Project
(from her book *An Altar of Words,* 1998)

CONTENTS

Acknowledgments xi

Foreword, *by M. Joycelyn Elders, M.D.* xiii

Introduction 1

    How to Use This Book 7

CHAPTER ONE: Was It Sexual Abuse? 11

    Help Yourself: Signs of Abuse? Questions to Ask 32

CHAPTER TWO: Overcoming Fear and Shame 34

    Help Yourself: Understanding Roots of Silence 49

CHAPTER THREE: Family Matters: Moving Beyond Denial 52

    Help Yourself: Creating the Space to Talk 75

CHAPTER FOUR: "Getting It Out" and Healing 77

    Help Yourself: African-Centered Healing 114

CHAPTER FIVE: Protecting and Saving Our Children 119

    Help Yourself: Become a Proactive Parent 145

CHAPTER SIX: Helping Boys and Men 149

    Help Yourself: Give Encouragement and Support 169

CHAPTER SEVEN: Challenging Abusers 172

    Help Yourself: Legal Issues and Finding a Lawyer 202

CHAPTER EIGHT: Reconciliation . . . and Moving On 204

    Help Yourself: Accountability and Responsibility 226

Resources 231

Notes 261

Bibliography 273

Index 277

ACKNOWLEDGMENTS

They say spirit moves, and there were days when I felt that spirit indeed was guiding my pen. For that sustaining force that makes all things possible, I am truly grateful.

No book is a solo effort. This one is the product of many. I want to thank those whose words and deeds have helped me throughout more than two years of research, reporting, and writing:

To the survivors who shared their remarkable stories, I am humbled by your trust in me, and encouraged by your fortitude.

To the many experts and healers who took the time to help me get it right.

To the circle of sisters who listened and listened and cheered me on: Dana Canedy, Georgia Scott, Deardra Griffin, Kimberly Perry, Carolyn Ellison, Katti Gray, and the Rev. Dr. Anne Elliott.

To my *Essence* family, past and present: Susan Taylor, for your continued inspiration; Patrik Bass, my muse, for helping me reach higher still; Monique Greenwood, for your sisterly spirit and open door at Akwaaba inns. To Ziba Kashef, asha bandele, Rosemarie Robotham, and Joan Morgan, for helping me get started. To Janice Bryant, for your superb editor's eye.

To my agent, Sarah Lazin, and my editor, Janet Hill, who believed in this book from Day 1, and the remarkable team at Doubleday/Broadway.

To Penny Duckham and colleagues at the Kaiser Family Foundation, for your generosity and support.

To Stacey Patton and Rozalynn Frazier, for your research and fine attention to detail; and to my niece Bridgette Bradford, who turned out a top-notch bibliography.

To my "readers" who were my extra eyes: Judith Zimmer, Penny Canedy, Maelinda Turner, and Dr. Dorothy Cunningham.

To Ora and Allen Hughes, my mom and stepfather, for your love and guidance.

To Terri Stone-Hill, for a lifetime of friendship and the brutal honesty that only a sister can provide.

To Gerald Boyd, my heart, for sharing yours with me. And to our amazing son, Zachary, whose fearlessness and free spirit remind me every day why I started down this path.

FOREWORD

by M. Joycelyn Elders, M.D.

Sexual abuse is a major public health problem, which is made more complex by the attitudes of our society in addressing issues involving sex.

We find it difficult to accept that offenders are often family members.

The act typically occurs in private, under a cloak of secrecy, and the nature of the act varies greatly in type, frequency, duration, and intensity. Since there may be no physical signs, sexual abuse is very difficult to detect.

Robin Stone's extraordinary book challenges the long-established wisdom of using myths, secrets, and lies to hide sexual abuse within a family circle. In a misguided attempt to maintain the bonds of a family group, people often try to minimize sexual abuse with expressions that tend to reduce the overwhelming consequences of the acts. Some of these expressions include "messin' with," "just playing," or "being warm and friendly." Ms. Stone sets us straight in *No Secrets, No Lies.*

She begins with her own story, describing how a child feels after sexual abuse—the fear, self-doubt, inability to come up with the right words to tell anyone. Then she narrates the stories of both women and men, focusing on incidents that happened when they were girls and boys. These heart-wrenching stories are told in an unsentimental way that touches us in their straightforwardness.

Learning the stories of others sometimes helps us not to feel so alone. When we realize that we are not solitary in our experience, we are more likely to delve into what has happened in our lives. Ms. Stone likens the yearning to "just put it behind us" to living with a persistent dental problem: "It doesn't go away—in fact, it gets worse. By the time you end up seeking help, you're in crisis."

She also explains how to help children avoid sexual abuse, as well as what to do and how to teach children how to respond if it should ever happen to them. She gives exact advice for adults who want to bring child sexual abusers to justice: how and where to find a lawyer, preparing for the visit to an attorney, and legal rights and limitations. She lists phone numbers, addresses and Web sites that can help you find the information you need.

Ms. Stone discusses what a family can do if there is a history of child sexual abuse, and she addresses some of the possibilities of outcomes. Three roads to resolution are presented: Confrontation, Accountability and Amends, Faith and Forgiveness. Exact actions and possible scenarios and words are given. While we all can sympathize with the problem, we do not all know what to do. The author delineates precisely how a survivor of sexual child abuse can rise out of the murky waters of secrets and lies.

Therapists, attorneys, clergy, and teachers as well as individuals who have been sexually abused as children who take Robin Stone's book to heart are likely to see a more accurate view of sexual child abuse and to experience gratifying personal growth.

As a society, we have a responsibility to protect children from sexual abuse. The most powerful weapon we have is *education*. This book will help us educate ourselves so that we can educate society and save the most valuable resource we will ever have—our children.

Dr. M. Joycelyn Elders, one of the nation's foremost advocates for comprehensive health education, including sex education, was U.S. Surgeon General in 1993–94.

NO SECRETS,
NO LIES

INTRODUCTION

If only this book weren't needed. But chances are that if you are reading it, you are seeking to help yourself or someone you love to heal from childhood sexual abuse. Know that you are not alone: an estimated one in four women and one in six men report that they were sexually abused as children.

I am among those survivors. For years I was also among the many who live in the shadows of silence and shame. Sexual abuse is a tough subject for most anyone to discuss, but it is especially difficult for those who have experienced it to expose long-buried wounds. For me, doing so took years of healing work, and in the end, it helped me see and understand not only the devastation of sexual violation, but also the damage of the silence, secrets, and denial that often follow.

Today, I am healthy and happy and whole. I have a husband and son whom I love dearly, family and friends whom I cherish, a spiritual center that keeps me grounded and helps me soar, a satisfying professional life, and meaningful connections with my community. But it wasn't easy to get there. Here's how I found my way.

I had been deputy editor of *Essence* magazine for about a year when, in 1998, our senior editorial team went on a retreat in upstate New York. The editor in chief at the time, Susan Taylor, had invited a motivational expert along to help us brainstorm for new article ideas.

Here we were, at the nation's leading magazine for Black women, gathered to find new ways to empower our readers. The expert started by asking each of us to draw two pictures—one as we saw ourselves, and the other as we'd like to see ourselves. When it was my turn, I held up my intricate handiwork: a harried-looking stick figure with disheveled hair struggling to balance two baskets of eggs, with some eggs spilling and others a cracked mess on the floor.

It was a reflection of my life as a wife and new mother, with a fairly new job and responsibilities as a new executive board member of a national non-profit organization—or so I thought. As I showed my second drawing, a serene, smiling sister, hair in place, calmly holding only one basket of neatly nestled eggs, I described my ideal life: less stress, fewer eggs, fewer demands. More time for me. And I added, offhandedly, that I hate dropping my eggs because I'm such a perfectionist. It stemmed, I said, from a memory of a relative telling me, when I eagerly showed off my report card with all A's and B's, "You still ain't shit." "I've been trying to prove them wrong ever since," I said.

I suddenly remembered how those words only confirmed what I had long felt: that no matter how hard I tried, I couldn't make up for a nagging sense of inadequacy. And quietly, to my surprise, I began to cry. At first, those tears annoyed me. *I'm a leader,* I remember thinking. *Leaders don't break down and cry in front of their colleagues.* But the more I thought about it, the more I realized that the first "me" drawing was a reflection of how I'd always lived: deeply immersed in everything—whether family or my work or my sorority or some other organization. I was always doing something *to keep from holding still.* I felt as if I was a voyeur in what seemed to be a perfect life, and I was tired of working so hard to avoid what really ailed me.

What I thought really ailed me was a severe lack of confidence. It became even more pronounced whenever I took on a major challenge, and at the time of that retreat, several major challenges were converging. Despite a stellar resume listing major accomplishments at some of the nation's best newspapers and magazines, despite successfully running a nonprofit organization, despite a new husband and baby, I always felt I was perpetrating a fraud, that I didn't deserve the achievements or even the joy in my life. At home, I would rarely relax, and work was all-encompassing. I would go in early, stay late, skip lunch, hover over my computer for so long that my neck and shoulders ached. I rarely gave myself credit for being smart and creative and passionate, for thinking fast and leading and always striving to do the right thing. That lack of confidence was my Achilles' heel, and that relative's remark had kept it tender over the years. From time to time I would try to shore it up by working on the symptoms but not the disease. Assertiveness-training courses, public-speaking courses, management courses, skills-development workshops, leadership seminars, you name it. I polished my presentations and buffed my skills to the point where I seemed to brim with confidence. But I couldn't shake those feelings of not measuring up.

All along, I knew that what really ailed me was a profound sense of shame and embarrassment that had been a part of my life for years. I'd often think: *There's something wrong with me, and I have to make up for it. There must be something wrong, because he chose me.*

I was a precocious kid in the early 1970s, the older of two girls raised by a single mother in a working-class section of northwest Detroit. Mom somehow found the time and money from her job at the post office to allow my sister and me to enjoy dance lessons and Saturday bowling and summertime softball. I loved writing and dancing and singing in the school chorus. Family reunions would find me front and center in our all-kid talent revues.

Children were abundant in our sprawling but tight-knit clan; cousins often spent the night at one house or another. Mom never thought for a moment that her kids wouldn't be safe.

When I was about nine, my sister and I slept over with family in the country. There, an uncle whom I adored led me by the hand to a back room and rubbed my breasts and between my legs. The incident, as I now refer to it, lasted about five minutes. But it left an impact that I still contend with today.

Messin' with. Touching. Fondling. Groping. Molesting. Incest. Abuse. Assault. Rape. I did not know the words for what happened to me that night with my uncle as the rest of the family slept. Often when we think of being sexually attacked, we see the culprit as someone who pounces from the bushes, not someone who tucks us in. We think of broken bones, or scars, or blood. If there is no visible, physical injury, it can be difficult to see that a deliberate crossing of the boundaries of appropriate behavior is indeed a form of violence.

All I knew is that when my uncle touched me, it didn't feel right. I also knew, literally knew, that what had happened was wrong when he told me not to tell. If nobody could know, it must have been bad. And by extension, I thought, I must have been bad. With the offer of a few dollars, my uncle told me to keep it a secret. I didn't take the money, but I made his secret mine and carried it for more than ten years. My mother became severely ill not too long after I was molested, and as she spent months on a slow, painful process of recovery, I tried in my child's way to take care of the trauma that I had suffered so that I wouldn't burden her. I would attend family gatherings and carefully avoid my uncle, fighting the waves of embarrassment whenever he would try to strike up a conversation with me as if nothing had ever happened. Many holiday get-togethers are a blur to me today; my time at them was consumed not with enjoying my family but with a vigilant act of keeping a safe distance from the enemy—my uncle—while watching to make sure he didn't take my younger sister off into some room.

I was confused and ashamed, and I felt isolated and alone, as no one else seemed to notice my distress.

I learned to take care of myself, but I wasn't always my best ally. I reasoned that I should never do anything to invite attention because I might be "chosen" again. So I became quiet and withdrawn. The girl who once sang on the stage and danced and laughed began to hide in the shadow of a hideous secret. I even hid in plain view: One summer I wore a red windbreaker nearly every day to cover up my growing breasts. I became a model student, striving for perfection to make up for my perceived imperfections. My little girl's mind told me that my uncle had picked me because he knew I was stupid enough to go along with him. I repeated that to myself so much that it rang true.

For years that secret weighed me down. I remember believing that I had done something to deserve what happened, and even as I wrestled with the meaning of what had happened, I sometimes managed to convince myself that it was really no big deal. *It only happened once,* I'd say to myself, minimizing the experience. I now know why sometimes we are reluctant to see an assault that's sexual in nature as violence. The majority of sexual abuse survivors know their offenders, and abusers operate so smoothly and convincingly that they gain the trust of children without the use of force. And as so many survivors do, I allowed my life to be shaped by a secret that wasn't mine to bear.

If I had known that my uncle had no right to touch me and that I could tell on him, then I might have yelled or screamed that night. If I had known then that our society and our own Black culture conspire to keep children quiet and vulnerable and Black women quiet and exploited, I would have been able to throw his secret back in his face. If I had known how we as a people are still struggling with the crippling effects of slavery and racism, I would have understood that my family's silence after the secret came out was nothing personal. It was inspired by years of fear and oppression and passed on from one generation to the next.

But I didn't have a clue. There were unspoken rules in my family and "around the way"—rules I learned from watching others around me. I knew to respect, not question or challenge my elders. I knew that some stuff you just didn't air in mixed company. I knew that breasts and hips were acceptable objects for commentary, especially from boys and men. I was self-conscious about my newly forming curves. Maybe I'd asked for that uncle's attention by wearing my favorite short shorts, I reasoned. Maybe I'd tempted him by sitting on his lap. What's a nine-year-old to think? For that matter, what's a three-year-old or a sixteen-year-old to think when someone she loves, respects, trusts, and perhaps even fears uses those feelings against her?

You may find it difficult to understand how five minutes can forever affect the course of a life. Or you may see yourself in some part of my story. Those who have been sexually abused know all too well the residue of shame and helplessness that the experience leaves behind. Few of us can imagine the complex network of scars that sexual abuse can create—whether it is one touch or a number of intricate "games" or years of intercourse. For me, I only knew that I needed teachers and family and friends to tell me I was smart and make me feel that I mattered. And whenever I had the nerve to think so myself, that nine-year-old girl would emerge to remind me to think again.

When I was twenty-one and preparing to move to Boston and brave the world on my own, I finally told my mother and stepfather after they gently encouraged me to explain why I refused to go to my uncle's house for my own going-away party. My mother was supportive and calm, at least in front of me. She called her sister, my aunt, to share what I had told her. The uncle, of course, said I was lying. My parents were left to choose whom to believe. They chose me. After some heated exchanges, my mother told a few other people in the family, and that uncle was told not to come around whenever I would be present. Mothers quietly asked their daughters if the uncle had ever "bothered" them. No one else said he did. No one spoke to me again about what had happened, and whenever the family gathered after that, my uncle simply was not there.

I was so relieved that the secret was out, but I didn't realize until later the damage I suffered. The abuse, the silence, and the survival skills I learned as a result played a major role in shaping my personality and my habits today. Without professional help back then, I dealt with the repercussions on my own. I grew up with few girlfriends because I felt "different" and older than most kids my age, and I found it difficult to open up and trust. It was easier to spend time with boys, and later men, because responding to physical attraction was easier than developing and nurturing relationships. Sex with no commitment was OK, I reasoned in my younger, single years, because I was in control of whom I slept with. In reality, I was being used and robbed of pieces of myself. And all the while, whenever I found the time to be still, I'd feel the unsettling sense of shame creeping upon me. Keeping busy kept it at bay. For a long time I knew there was something wrong, but again, I focused on the symptoms and not the cause.

One time, about ten years ago, I tried to fix the symptoms. Citing stress and anxiety, I went to see a therapist I picked out of my insurance company's directory. We never got to the abuse. Whenever I talked about anything related to race, the therapist, who was White, would stare at me blankly. I remember telling her how painful it was to hear a White male newspaper colleague tell me that my ignorance of an obscure grammatical rule was the result of poor education. I should have been angry, yet I thought of my public schooling and heard that nine-year-old's voice say, *See? I told you you were stupid,* and I went home feeling defeated not by him but by myself. The therapist could offer nothing to counter my sense of humiliation, obviously not sensitive to the struggles of Blacks in White corporate America. I didn't stick around for long.

That day at the retreat, when the facilitator encouraged us to talk about our stress, I looked into the faces of my colleagues, Black women of all hues and shapes and sizes, and saw in their eyes that they understood just what it meant to work too hard, to juggle too much, to stretch too thin in search of perfection. In the cocoon of that sister circle, I felt comfortable enough to let my guard down, and the tears came from years of being tired and ashamed. Another sister cried too. Susan Taylor put her arm around my shoulder and reminded me, "We're so glad you're with us—you bring us so much." It was a compliment that I allowed myself to believe. Later I asked a coworker to recommend a good Black therapist for me to see.

It took twenty-five years for me to understand how five minutes of horror, in the shadow of a relative's house, could affect my life so deeply. I found a new therapist, a Black woman who understood my experience with corporate racism and who made me feel as if I was talking to a friend. With her help, I started to unravel the secret and feelings of shame and self-doubt from my life.

As I began to heal, I searched everywhere for information about abuse within families—Black families in particular. I wanted to know about the many fears that keep us quiet, and how race colored our perspective. In candid talks with my mother, I explored how abuse affected our own family. We had a predator among us, but no one seemed to know what else to do about my violation, or his abnormal, criminal behavior, so they simply made him stay away. It was clear that we all needed help. I set out to find it.

I started with a trip to the library, then I visited some Web sites and talked to friends. Almost as soon as I would tell them about my research, many quietly shared their own painful experiences with sexual abuse. I was struck by how merely raising the topic helped them open up. My research led to an article in *Essence* about how speaking out about past abuse can bring healing. The article explained how sexual abuse, and the silence that surrounds it, affects our physical and mental well-being, how it shapes our lives and influences the choices we make. In response, I received more than five hundred e-mails, letters, and phone calls, many of them from people sharing their stories for the first time. Several are featured in the chapters that follow.

In searching for books to read about healing from the trauma of childhood sexual abuse, I came across many useful guides and personal accounts (they are listed in the Resources section, page 231). But none spoke to my need as a Black woman, a survivor, and a journalist to understand sexual abuse within Black families, and the impact of abuse on our lives and the lives of those who are closest to us. Why do family members blame the victims, for instance, or why do survivors keep quiet "for the sake of the family"? As I gathered the answers, I knew I had the makings of a book.

No Secrets, No Lies is for those who want a way to explain what nobody knows how to voice. It is for those who hope never to have to help a loved one through such a painful experience. It is for those who are looking for a way to stop feeling "ugly, dirty, worthless," as Debra, a survivor, wrote to me. It is for those who are looking to say, "This happened to me" and "It was not my fault." It is for those who want justice but never knew how to find it. It is about our families, our history, our culture, and our "issues," told in our voices, held up as a mirror that helps us see even what we don't want to.

HOW TO USE THIS BOOK

No Secrets, No Lies is separated into three main parts: background on child sexual abuse, powerful personal stories from survivors and their family members, and practical, easy-to-follow guidance from experts who work with and treat survivors and abusers. "Fast Facts"—most of which help convey the scope of the problem in general and among African Americans in particular—appear throughout.

One of the best ways to learn is by example, so you will gain that knowledge in the following chapters—with the help of dozens of courageous women and men who have shared with me their own inspiring stories of abuse, survival, and healing. I start by clarifying what sexual abuse is and how big this problem is. Then I explore why we don't see abuse even when it's staring us in the face. I also show how our society allows and even encourages physical and sexual violence, especially against women and children. And I identify those attitudes and behaviors that we've inherited from our culture, our parents, and even our ancestors that allow abuse to happen in our families and that keep us from getting help when we need it.

I interviewed more than thirty survivors, along with mothers, fathers and other family members. Because of their sensitive nature, I conducted most of my interviews in person, in the privacy of homes or the anonymity of quiet restaurants. I traveled to fifteen cities and visited a prison, an elementary school, a church, a drug treatment center for women, and a treatment center for sexual abusers. Through a one-way mirror, I watched as survivors challenged sexual abusers and batterers in a therapy session.

For many of the people I spoke with, talking about "family business" wasn't easy. For so many of us, it's just not our way. But their stories give us a window into how family members have handled sexual abuse in their lives, and how survivors have managed to do just that—survive—because of, or in spite of, their families. The people I interviewed are no different from you or me. They go to jobs every day, they pay their taxes, give their tithes, rear their children. Many of them agreed to talk to me simply because they felt they could help others. Their experiences mirror the conflict and anguish typical of families dealing with abuse.

A humbled mother and father speak candidly about how, twenty years later, they finally came to acknowledge that their daughter had been molested by her grandfather. A sister shares her shame and embarrassment over her brother's abuse of his stepdaughter. A mother tells of her struggle to help her daughter, the abused, and not forsake the son, the abuser. A wife speaks of the love she still has for her husband, who is in prison for abusing her daughter. You will meet survivors who ran away, who scarred their bodies, who tried to take their lives. And through their stories, you will see the relentless toll of abuse, the strength and resilience of those who confront their past, and the many ways that you can move on with your life.

I explain how sexual abuse and the silence that accompanies it reverberate far beyond the survivor and abuser, and how those reverberations can last for years. Unchecked, they strike at the very core of a survivor—damaging self-esteem, causing depression, limiting potential—but they can also undermine what should be a critical source of strength and support: family. I detail how abusers operate, what makes them tick, and how they can be stopped. And I share how to protect our kids and how to help if they are abused. I've gathered the most widely accepted holistic and traditional healing practices and show how each can help and how some work together.

In the personal stories, you will meet many who have overcome or are working to overcome sexual abuse. You will hear from the families and a partner of those who've been abused, and abusers themselves. To protect their privacy and as a legal precaution (few accused of abuse in these instances have been charged with or convicted of a crime), names and some identifying details of those interviewed have been changed. But know that I've rendered their stories just as they were described.

The following experts offer advice to help you or someone you love: leading psychologists, social workers, lay counselors, spiritual advisers, activists, and holistic healers nationwide. They show us how to apply to our own lives the lessons we learn from survivors' stories. Each chapter is followed by a section called "Help Yourself," interactive quizzes, writing, and other exercises provided by or developed with the help of experts. They will give you further insight into yourself or your situation. Keep a journal handy to explore your thoughts and feelings. Listings at the end of the book point you to the right resources and services.

It is my hope that *No Secrets, No Lies* will inspire and educate. That survivors connect with the personal stories and follow the experts' advice. That counselors and advisers see new ways to help their clients. And that family and friends gain a deeper understanding of the extent and trauma of sexual abuse. Perhaps this is the beginning of a conversation that you didn't know how to start. Or your way of helping someone you know is hurting. You may not agree with everything here, and you may find some stories too painful to read. But know that sexual abuse is a difficult subject for all too many to face, and that you have taken an enormous step forward in trying to understand it.

Put this book to use. Take what you need to help yourself and others. Do the exercises. Share the stories. Speaking truth to power is the only way to end the secrets and lies that we have carried for generations. It is the only way to protect our children and begin to mend our families.

The survivors' stories that I share represent a patchwork quilt of real-life approaches to dealing with and ending child sexual abuse. You will find that there is no simple solution to how Black families can heal from this very private violation that has enormous public costs. In fact, some families need to be fractured before they can heal. The most common threads between each richly detailed quilt piece is the strength and resilience of survivors and the determination of each to stop the cycle of abuse. That, in and of itself, is a soul-satisfying step toward healing. Let's take that first step together.

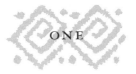

ONE

Was It Sexual Abuse?

I just didn't think that adults had sex with children.

DARLENE, who as a preteen was raped
repeatedly by a brother-in-law

I F YOU ARE READING THIS BOOK, YOU MIGHT HAVE FOUND AT SOME point in your life that you were on your own, searching for the words to name what was happening to you. Or for the courage to get away, or the power to make it stop. You may have figured that it happened to everybody, because it had become so routine in your life. You might have even expected it, felt your body respond to it. You might have carried the secret for years, or maybe you're still carrying it today.

Without enlightenment, we struggle, we are on our own, in the dark, trying to understand why we're "evil, all the time," as one sister said to me. Or why our families may get together and laugh easily but rarely come to terms with deep, deep troubles. For many of us, we have buried sexual abuse so deep into our psyches that we would never connect it to today's physical illnesses and pain, our depression or addiction, our inability to hold a job, get out of debt, find satisfaction in a relationship, nurture our children, or simply say no to people or situations that do us harm.

But knowledge, as does faith, helps to light the way. Knowledge clears the fog of ignorance so that we can see what's real and true, even if it's ugly. It helps us see how our families enable and even encourage abuse. And it helps us learn how to hold abusers accountable, or at the least not be intimidated by them. Knowledge helps us understand how abuse has affected our lives and what we can do to untangle those effects from the life we want to live. And it helps us see our experience within the context of our culture and the larger society.

ALL ABOUT POWER

Sexual abuse, simply put, is when a person in power or authority uses you or forces you to perform for his or her sexual gratification. Sexual abuse can range from noncontact flashing and use of explicit pictures and language to touching and kissing to digital and penile penetration. It is a crime, which often stems from a sickness.[1] And it is a violation of your body, your mind, and your spirit. It is perhaps the nature of the crime that leads us to believe that what happens behind closed doors should stay there, but it is often in the shadow of silence that problems like depression and addiction develop, enabling abuse to continue for generations.

The power of an abuser can be physical or assumed. Clergy members and teachers have power in their positions as spiritual and educational leaders. A friend of the family has power because he is an adult and because he has connections to the parents that a child does not have. The power of a boss or coach stems from that role of authority. A babysitter's power and authority are inherent in her position as a caregiver and substitute for parents. A cousin may not be bigger in size but may seem to have more household clout because of the way he commands his elders' attention and respect. The term *incest* can mean sexual relations between family members, regardless of age. Throughout my book I will use the terms *child sexual abuse* and *sexual abuse,* which more specifically describes adults' illegal sexual contact with children.

I will focus on the sexual abuse of children and abuse committed by family, informal family, and friends because we are more likely to be abused as children than as adults, and, contrary to the "stranger danger" warnings that many of us remember from childhood, we are most likely to be abused by someone we know.[2] It is in these instances—in a tangle of confusion, fear, embarrassment, and shame—that the silence is most pervasive. Most abuse is committed by adult males against younger females, though women are known to abuse, children are known to abuse, and boys and young men are also abused.[3] I will refer most often to instances in which women were abused in childhood by adult males, but I have included a chapter (Chapter 6) on the specific challenges of boys who are abused.

If you have ever been sexually abused, then you should consider yourself a survivor in recognition of your fortitude, no matter the negative impact, no matter what harmful ways you have found to cope with your experience. Anyone who has been sexually violated and has lived to tell about it, including myself, I will refer to as a survivor. I give a nod to the noted feminist scholar Traci C. West, who uses the term *victim-survivor* to remind readers "of the dual status of women who have been victimized by assault and survived it." She notes: "Black women are sometimes denied an opportunity to have their victimization recognized."[4]

A survivor once wrote to me: "Is it abuse if you don't have sex?" The answer is: Absolutely. We might dismiss or minimize our experience of abuse because it was "only touching" or "it happened only once" or "it was a long time ago." But abuse has many forms and faces, and each can be devastating in its own way. You can determine if what you experienced was abuse by asking yourself these questions:

What Happened?

- Was I touched or kissed in a way that made me feel uncomfortable?
- Were words with sexual overtones used to describe my body?
- Were words about sexual acts used in my presence?
- Was I made to view sexual acts?
- Was I made to pose for sexual photos or movies?
- Was I forced to touch someone else's genitals or breasts?
- Was I made to put my mouth on someone else's genitals or breasts?
- Was I raped or penetrated?
- Was the person who did this in a more powerful role than me (bigger, stronger, older, in authority)?

If you answered yes to any of these questions, you were most likely sexually abused. The "Help Yourself" exercise at the end of this chapter focuses on the symptoms that can help you acknowledge past abuse. Together these questions and the exercise can help you be clear and sure. It doesn't matter how long ago, or how often, though more severe abuse has been linked to more severe health-related problems.[5] One episode is enough to cause a lifetime of damage. There need not be a threat or physical violence, merely a touch, innuendo, or some other sexual act that makes you uncomfortable. And without some form of therapeutic help, it is difficult to simply "get over it," as many survivors are told to do, or have tried to do. Shirley, who is in her seventies, still vaguely remembers being abused by her mother's husband, a man whom she refuses to call "father." She was about three at the time it started. Whenever she speaks out about it, she finds that through her testimony, she heals a bit more: "My daily life is not fraught with fear. But the triggers, they take me back to where I was. Triggers like what's happening with the Catholic Church and all those priests, or somebody might touch me when I'm not expecting it. I've not done all my work in healing. I've done it in segments over the years. And I've learned to tell my story. I've just tried to get functional. That's good enough for me."

HOW BIG IS THIS PROBLEM?

Because of fear, shame, and cultural baggage, most of us keep this violation to ourselves, making sexual abuse one of the least-reported crimes in the United States.[6] Statistics vary widely, depending on the type of research and the size of the study's sample, and even what behaviors are considered abusive. About 87,000 children were sexually abused in 2001, according to the Department of Health and Human Services' National Child Abuse and Neglect Data System, which tracks confirmed cases of abuse. But chronic underreporting means that no statistics truly reflect the extent of abuse in our country. These widely quoted numbers from surveys of adults looking back on their childhoods reflect how prevalent the problem is: About one in four women and one in six men report that they were sexually abused as children.[7]

Using these estimates, among African Americans, that translates to about 3.3 million women and 1.9 million men eighteen and older who have reported a history of sexual abuse.[8] If it were considered a disease, experts would have labeled sexual abuse an epidemic long ago.

Comprehensive research on sexual abuse is relatively new; major studies on the issue have been produced only in the last twenty or so years. And not surprisingly, research that focuses on Black Americans' experience is rare; few studies examine the role of race and culture in survivors' experiences. One noted exception is the work of Gail E. Wyatt, a clinical psychologist and professor at UCLA. I will refer regularly to Wyatt's pioneering in-depth studies exploring the impact of abuse on the lives of Black women. "We're certainly not the only group that's silent regarding abuse," says Wyatt, who has written several books on abuse and sexuality. "But we're the only group whose experience is compounded by our history of slavery and stereotypes about Black sexuality, and that makes discussion more difficult."

Abuse is debilitating. Its impact on behavior is lifelong and potentially deadly. For children, abuse can stunt their psychological and emotional development. E. Sue Blume writes that abused children experience "a course of development (emotional, interpersonal, sexual) that is shared, every day, with premature sexuality, lack of safety (even terror) and deformities of many life skills. The child victim's entire view of herself and the world will be clouded by the effects of her abuse."[13]

Most research into sexual abuse focuses on the psychological effects: Survivors are more likely to experience depression than women who weren't abused, studies show; the longer the abuse lasts and the more violent, the more severe the problems.[14] However, no study can truly reflect the range of experiences and their related effects. One woman who was propositioned but never touched by her mother's boyfriend spoke of an enormous sense of shame that she was somehow enticing him. We will explore the impact of abuse, and the silence that often follows, in the next two chapters.

Many psychological problems can lead to or complicate physical problems, such as reproductive disorders. Abuse also affects women's sexual choices: Survivors are more likely to engage in risky sexual behavior that leads to disease and pregnancy. In one study, 66 percent of pregnant teens

Fast Facts

- Blacks are sexually victimized in childhood at the same rate as Whites. In one survey, they reported being more severely abused with greater force.[9]
- Family members and acquaintances account for 93 percent of sexual assaults against people under age eighteen.[10]
- In estimates of cases known to child protective agencies or community workers, girls were sexually abused three times more often than boys.[11]
- Sexual abuse before age eighteen increases a woman's risk of becoming HIV-positive more than any other factor in her life.[12]

reported a history of abuse.[15] Sixty-six percent of all prostitutes were sexually abused as children, and 66 percent of sexually abused prostitutes were abused by fathers, stepfathers, or foster fathers.[16] Another recent study showed that sexual abuse before age eighteen increased a woman's risk of becoming HIV-positive more than any other factor in her life.[17]

Ultimately, as a society, we all pay for sexual abuse through public and private money spent on crisis intervention, child protection services, medical treatment, foster care, and the criminal justice system. Other directly related costs include those for mental health care and counseling, substance abuse treatment, and social services programs for indigent clients and the mentally ill. Among secondary costs, consider simply the cumulative lost time from work that can be linked to survivors' history of sexual violation. Studies have shown that it is far cheaper to provide prevention services than to pay for intervention and treatment.

All acts of sexual abuse should be reported immediately to your local police, rape crisis center, or social service agency, and the survivor should get immediate physical and mental help. By law, adults whose work puts them in contact with children are supposed to report signs that a child has been abused (see Chapter 5, "Protecting and Saving Our Children") to the authorities. In some states, every person with a reasonable suspicion must report or face fines or even jail time. Adult survivors who want to take legal action against their abusers may do so by pressing criminal charges or filing a civil lawsuit. Whatever the judicial outcome of the abuser's case, that person must receive professional treatment as well. We will explore treatment for survivors and reporting abusers in Chapters 4 and 7.

WHY IS THIS *OUR* PROBLEM?

Sexual abuse spans all racial, gender, economic, and social boundaries. At least one study shows that abuse is more common among children in lower-income families.[18] Because African Americans are disproportionately poor, it may seem that Blacks are at a disproportionate risk for being abused. But it should be noted that abuse is more likely *to be reported* among low-income families because they tend to be in contact with public agencies and authorities more than others, and may be observed more. Also, those who tend to report suspicions of abuse, such as teachers and doctors, may be more likely to suspect abuse in lower-income families. That means that the problem goes virtually undetected in those families whose race or ethnicity, money, status, or social standing insulates them from people who might otherwise turn a trained eye to warning signs.

Abuse is our problem because while studies show that Black children are victimized just as often as White children, survivors report different reactions to their experiences. And we must remember that in addition to the trauma of sexual violation, survivors must also deal with the trauma of being born and raised in a racist and sexist culture.[19] Wyatt's study comparing experiences of rape includes some significant differences:[20]

- Black American women were more likely to have withheld reports of attempted rape from authorities.
- Black Americans were significantly more likely than Whites to blame their living circumstances for placing them at risk for victimization.
- Black Americans tended to be the victims of repeated assaults slightly more often than Whites.
- Black Americans were significantly more likely than Whites to have heard sexual and racial stereotypes regarding which kinds of women are likely to be raped.

In another study, Blacks reported that they were more likely than Whites to be abused severely in terms of the sex acts involved, and the abuse was more likely to be accompanied by force. They were less likely to be abused by a father and more often abused by their uncles.[21] I will show in detail in this and the following chapters some specific ways that Black women were affected.

HOW WE LET ABUSE HAPPEN

Most of us take for granted the requirements for belonging to a family, if we've given it any thought at all. Perhaps if we had to sign a contract, we'd be forced to acknowledge the awesome responsibilities that come with being a part of a clan.

Every family has an unspoken trust. It's the assumption that kin should be a source of nurturing, sharing, and safety. Unfortunately, not all of our families provide all of these things, but each family member at least has a responsibility to keep its children safe. That extends to nieces and nephews, cousins and beyond. Our children don't ask to be here, as my mother solemnly reminded me when my son was born. We have a moral and even legal obligation to care for them until they are old enough to care for themselves.

But care goes far beyond the physical needs that quickly come to mind: food, clothing, shelter. Care means tending to their emotional needs, too. It means honoring them and respecting their rights (See "The Child's Bill of Rights," page 148). It means knowing their likes and dislikes, what scares them, what delights them. It means embracing them and listening to them and letting them know that nothing is more important than what they have to say. To do anything less is to do harm. Gail Wyatt cites studies that connect a lack of maternal warmth with low self-esteem and suggests that children with low self-esteem may be more likely to be chosen as targets by molesters and less successful in fending off assault.[22]

Sexual abuse is a violation of that unspoken family trust, as one author describes.[23] And when we look the other way or don't call out a situation of abuse, then we too are breaking the family trust. We often think that abuse involves only the victim and the abuser. That's why it is so easy for some to turn away, saying, "Not my problem." But when abuse occurs, all family members in some way are either victims, perhaps because they too are afraid to face the secret, or victimizers, because they are in denial.[24]

If abuse occurs in a family that is already coping with its own problems, be they personal, economic, social, or legal, then the situation is further complicated because the family is focused on other priorities and communication is rare or nonexistent. As my interviews with survivors show time and time again, adults often are simply not aware of their children's needs. Typically they know something is not quite right, but they say or do nothing because of fear and denial. For twenty years, Allen didn't acknowledge that his daughter had been abused by her paternal grandfather. In explaining why, Allen put it this way: "I could justify it because Maya was so manipulative in those days. So it was convenient for me to say, 'That's just another wild story.' It took me off the hook from pursuing anything."

Maybe our kids are so hungry for nurturing that abuse looks like love to them. Maybe we're not talking and listening to them enough. Maybe some adult is paying too much attention to them and parents are too preoccupied to see the warning signs. If abuse is not properly addressed and treated, it can sow the seeds of further dysfunction. The secrets and lies keep us from developing and nurturing open relationships with one another, and keep abuse survivors from living fully. Families come to know one another—and the world—through a veil of deception.

We may be the epitome of the Joneses, living high on the hill, or Joe and Josephine Public, struggling to get out of the projects and off welfare. Doesn't matter. If we allow a space for our children to be vulnerable and then turn our eyes from their signs of distress, abusers can strike in our homes, under our noses. And as you will see from the following story, our children will be at great risk.

DARLENE'S STORY:
"HOW COULD THEY NOT HAVE KNOWN?"

Darlene, who lives in Philadelphia, speaks and writes with the wisdom of a woman far beyond her twenty-six years. As a counselor in the city's public schools, she's familiar with families who are homeless, who live in shelters, whose parents are so strung out on some substance that they forget to take their kids to class. As she looks back on her preteen years, a time when she was repeatedly raped by a brother-in-law, she sees that in some ways, her own family was much like those she now works with.

Darlene was the baby, the youngest of a dozen brothers and sisters. The family lived in a rambling old row house with an apartment in the basement. Younger kids lived upstairs, and older ones stayed downstairs until they were old enough to move out. It was a large and extended family, with an occasional cousin joining them for a year or so at a time. It was always busy, she remembers. "Always somebody coming and going and always something going on."

Darlene grew up with four sisters, but although the girls depended on one another, she says, "I never felt close to any of them." The girls were all a year or two apart, then came lots of boys. Darlene's was a church-going family: most Tuesdays, Fridays, Saturdays, and Sundays you could find them at a Methodist service or event.

Her father, a trucker, was on the road at least six months out of the year. "I always felt like my mother was working, my father wasn't there," she remembers. "We weren't really close to him. It was, 'Hi, Dad, when are you leaving again?'" He was strict and neat, while her mother, a nurse, was the opposite. "When Dad was home, we'd have breakfast together. When Mom was home, we could eat in our room."

Darlene was on her own. "You'd think there were lots of people to talk to, but no," she says. "I always had food, I always had a home, and I was the littlest, so I got attention. But it was not, 'What's going on in your life? How's school?'"

When she was eleven, one of her sisters was living in the basement with her husband. The sister was nineteen and her husband, twenty-three. They were expecting their second child. One night as Darlene slept in the room she shared with another sister, her brother-in-law came in, woke her, and led her to a bathroom. "It was dark and cold," she recalls. "He said: 'You know, Stacy's pregnant, and I need for you to do me a favor. If you help me with this, I'll get you whatever you want.' And I thought of a red bike. And so he turned me around, and pulled down my shorts, and did it right there in the bathroom."

Darlene doesn't remember much else from that night, except the pain and the questions. "I just stood there, just stood there with my hands like this," she says, imitating the way her hands were pressed high against the wall. "And then it was like, 'Thank you, don't tell anybody.' I didn't cry or say anything. I just remember my head felt hot—I think I was shocked. I had never heard of it. I just didn't think that adults had sex with children. I remember going back to my room thinking, *What happened? Why?*"

The rapes continued, two, maybe three nights a week, until Darlene was thirteen. Sometimes at night, sometimes in the day. Different places and different positions. He always offered to take her somewhere, to get her alone. Once, he fondled her on a bus. Darlene's mother worked the afternoon shift, leaving her home a lot. And sometimes other people were home. "My sister was in her bunk one time," she says. "How could they not have known? But then I found out later that he had tried it with my two other sisters, and they had said no. But instead of warning me, they just let it go."

When she was twelve, a schoolteacher gave a talk on sex abuse. Darlene called a hotline. They told her to tell someone, but she refused. "'He seems like a good guy with my sister,'" she remembers saying. "'This is the only problem that I see them having, and I don't want to mess that up for her.' I was really trying to keep him happy for her. I decided not to say anything."

Her mother suspected something was up with her daughter. She came to her one day and said, "I think I know what's happened, and I think I know who it is. And I want you to tell me, because I know somebody else it happened to."

Darlene immediately thought of her sisters, and how they refused him. And then she remembered that he had given her a few dollars to keep quiet. "I was so ashamed, so I said nothing happened. But she didn't believe me." Her mother put her brother-in-law out of the house and reported him to the police. But because Darlene would not change her story, the police had no case.

Darlene's sister moved out with her husband, "as if nothing had happened." Darlene was furious, and hurt. "I started to act out, running away from home, staying out late. I was out of control. I'd tell my sisters I hated them, and the sister with the husband, I hated her most of all." She sought out an older woman from church, writing her a letter describing the abuse. The woman called their pastor, who called Darlene's mother.

"They called a family meeting," Darlene remembers. "They were trying to get me to talk." But the meeting went nowhere. "One brother was saying I was crazy, and two other brothers started arguing, so I walked out," she says. "It seemed nobody cared about me. They just cared that I was acting out. I was angry that he was never punished. But I think I was more angry that they didn't look out for me."

Darlene stayed away from home more, "taking pills, drinking, cutting myself: my arms, my chest, and legs," she says. "I wanted to make myself look ugly, so guys wouldn't look at me." A few times, she tried to kill herself. One try landed her in a psychiatric hospital, where she began antipsychotic drugs. Once when she ran away, she was raped by a man she had met on the subway. "It was late and cold and I was tired of sleeping on the train," she says. "He offered to let me crash at his place. I've never told a soul about it until now. That one I felt really was my fault."

Darlene managed to graduate from high school and then college with honors. Perhaps in the chaos of her family, she saw school as a safe haven. Psychological counseling probably saved her life. "I realized that I had put a lot of the ownership on me. But my sister's husband was the adult and it was his fault."

She is not close to her family today. She lives with her mother, primarily to save money. They rarely speak.

It is not unusual that Darlene is a counselor, even though she still needs help herself. Some of the experts I have interviewed cite a history of abuse, and indeed suggest that they became counselors and activists because of their experience. Darlene has tried to move on, but she is still troubled by her past. "Things still bother me," she says. "There was nothing—no punishment, no apology. I'm depressed. And I mask it by keeping busy at the job, sleeping a lot. I don't eat well. I still drink. I usually sleep with the TV or the lights on. I guess I always feel like I'm going to be attacked. Like somebody's holding you down and you can't get up. Or you're screaming and you're not heard."

WHAT SOCIETY TELLS US

Darlene was a perfect target for an abuser. Not just because she was a child, but also because, in the swirl of humanity in her household, she was lost, and vulnerable, fending for herself. From her story, it is clear to see that she had also been conditioned to believe that she did not matter.

Sexual abuse does not happen in a vacuum. By our example, we adults teach children their roles in relationships and society. What they don't learn from us and other kids, they pick up from the media. The typical messages for our kids: that children are expendable, that men matter most, that Blacks are inferior. While positive messages can empower, consistently negative messages can nip away at an already fragile self-esteem. In Darlene's case, those family and cultural influences worked against her.

Darlene learned how to be used. She learned that adults' needs were more important than hers. She learned that the only way to get the attention of her family was to disrupt it by "acting out." She learned that she was somehow a partner in the abuse, and that she deserved whatever she got.

These are among the cultural messages that make children like Darlene easy targets for abuse:

- **Children's needs come last.** Many of us grew up with the message that children should be seen and not heard, and that there is a definite pecking order: men's needs are satisfied first, women come next, and children are last. With this thinking, it is no wonder that Darlene felt it was her obligation to do "favors" for her sister's husband, to "keep him happy." Darlene believed that others' needs were more important than hers.

- **There's no time or place for problems.** If children aren't the priority, they quickly learn, neither are their worries and fears. "Many parents are unconscious to their children's needs," says noted self-help author Brenda Richardson. "It doesn't mean that you don't feed your children—that you don't keep a roof over them. It means the welcome mat isn't out when it comes to sharing how you're feeling." If you grew up in a home where your feelings didn't matter, Richardson suggests, then "the message was: 'We don't want to hear your problems. We want to hear you're doing well because, well, I have so much going on myself that I just can't handle any more problems.'" The result: children don't want to be a burden, and keep their pain to themselves.

- **Let's *not* talk about sex.** Many survivors remember being told that they were being "prepared" for relationships with men. "He told me that in different cultures, fathers did it with their daughters," Tracey, a thirty-year-old Chicago sister, says of her father, who repeatedly molested her for about ten years. And when children don't know about their body parts, how they function, and which ones are off-limits, they are more likely to believe that the "lessons" are for their own benefit, at least at first. We are flooded with images and references to sex—most of them negative—in a society that historically has been uptight about sexual expression and behavior. Faye Wattleton, long-time advocate for women's reproductive rights and president of the Center for Gender Equality, suggests that kind of combination leaves children vulnerable to countless negative cultural influences, countered by none from home. "Why is it easier to embrace an Eminem, for instance, than to have healthy sexuality conversation in schools and families?" asks Wattleton, former president of the Planned Parenthood Federation of America. "Why do we address sexuality in such a bizarre, perverse manner?" If we don't talk with our kids on our own terms, we leave them to sort out powerful cultural messages on their own, navigating the unpredictable and sometimes perilous terrain of sex without a roadmap that can keep them safe.

- **Boys will be boys, and girls will be weak.** Most boys are rewarded, or at least ignored, for being aggressive, while girls are encouraged to get along and "act like ladies." Girls keep peace and adapt, and boys take what they want. Our society does not value getting along as much as it does being first and fast, and winning. And it certainly does not value what are considered feminine characteristics. One of the worst insults you can hurl at a male is to say he acts "like a sissy" or plays "like a girl." Domestic violence experts Meg Kennedy Dugan and Roger Hock suggest that even the seemingly innocent message that fathers give their young sons to "take care of Mom while Dad's away" is loaded with meaning: that even as a child, a boy carries the burden of protector, and that he can expect to assume control over others, especially females. When girls are encouraged to be caretakers, it's not a matter of control, the experts say, but of sacrificing their own needs to tend to others.[25]

- **Women are opposite, not equal.** Until the early twentieth century, even White American women (and children) were considered men's property and had few legal rights. This social structure still influences our expectations of how men and women should behave. "Where men are seen as dominant, women are expected to be submissive," Kennedy Dugan and Hock assert. "Where men are active, women should be passive. Where men are in control, women should be willing to obey."[26] In relationships and child-rearing, many women still refer to men as "head of the household" instead of equal partners. These roles leave little room for women to feel they can take charge of their situations, especially if the men in their lives are controlling or domineering.

- **Don't ask, don't tell.** In a country in which the right to privacy is guaranteed by the Constitution, what goes on inside our homes is often seen as off-limits to scrutiny from outside. A clear violation of law against an outsider is likely to warrant a neighbor's call to the police, but when that violation calls for challenging a parent's authority over his or her children (as in cases of spankings or beatings), or challenging "consenting adults" (as in cases of domestic abuse), many people are reluctant to speak up. And certainly few want to get involved if the violation involves sex, which, in general, is socially taboo. As Faye Wattleton says: "The protection that is granted to the home enables the kind of power that is hard to breach. I worked most of my career to keep the government out of my life and my home, but that doesn't apply if I'm committing a crime."

- **Women exist for sexual pleasure.** Much of our popular music conveys this notion: lyrics present us first as reluctant participants who need to be coaxed into sex. If we give in and say yes, then we become receptacles, having things done to us, put in us, being "filled up." On videos, we're half-clothed or less, lips parted, breasts jiggling, thighs spread, bumping, grinding, decorations on the arms of a male center of attention. There may be two or more of us, all tending to one man.

- **It's the victim's fault.** From the Bible's portrayal of women as temptresses (remember Eve? Delilah?) to much of society's assumption that rape victims "ask" for it by way of their dress or behavior, women have always been blamed for encouraging sex. If women exist for men's sexual pleasure, the reasoning goes, women tease, and men aren't at fault for forcing them. This thinking is so ingrained that survivors may often blame themselves for the abuse they sustained. Traci West writes:

  > Women may believe that they should have fought harder or longer against their attacker. Children rarely fight their attackers as they are most often abused by those they already trust. . . . In almost every instance, self-blame centers around a woman's doubt of her own experience of violence. . . . The doubt is fueled by a mythical image of what an "authentic" victim "should" be. There are certain emotional reactions she "should" have had, and particular actions that she "should" have taken during an incident of violence. Failure to fulfill the expectations within this mythical scenario means that she shares responsibility for her ordeal. [27]

- **Violence against women is normal.** As many experts agree, violence is simply a by-product of our male-dominated society. "In most feminist discussions of violence against women, it is assumed that men assault women because they can," West writes. This is not because of physical might, but a social assumption: "Male violation of women is a 'right' possessed by all men in our society." [28] Even most religious teachings tell us that the man is the head of the household, and our spiritual communities have been known to look the other way when that position is enforced by fear or force. Mass media further this presumption. When a jilted man kills a woman, the crime is often described as one of "passion." The implication is that the killer is excused to some degree because of the "passion" that gripped him while he was taking her life. Think about it: Even popular language describing sexuality often refers to power, conquest, and violence. If language is a mirror of a culture, Kennedy Dugan and Hock suggest, the words we use reflect our views of men, women, and sex:

Consider some common English slang for male and female sexual anatomy: Words such as "tool," "manhood," and "sword" to refer to the penis suggest power, strength, and even dangerous weapons. However, slang used for female anatomy . . . often includes terms that suggest something passive, a non-active receptacle. "Hole," "tunnel," "honey pot" are common examples. More disturbing are colloquialisms describing female sexual anatomy as victimized by the male "weapon." "Gash," "slit" are such terms. . . . Words such as banging, screwing, nailing (as in "he nailed her") suggest that intercourse is not a mutual, loving event but an act involving varying degrees of aggression that the man perpetrates on the woman. [29]

WHAT ENSLAVEMENT LEFT US

Sexual abuse can happen no matter what our social standing or race. And even though African Americans are a richly diverse people, spanning the spectrum of lifestyles and interests, education, income, religious background, and extent of assimilation, because of our unique legacy of slavery, racism, and oppression, we've inherited some common, profoundly destructive behaviors that blind us, keep us silent, leave the victim vulnerable, and leave the victimizer free to continue to abuse. These behaviors only compound the negative influences from the larger society, making our children especially easy prey.

That our people survived 250 years in bondage is a testament to their strength and resilience. Eight generations of families born in servitude, their very existence at the whim of White masters. Property, bought and sold, bred, beaten, and worked to death. Slaveholders systematically chipped away at our dignity, our humanity, and our knowledge of our own histories and languages and cultures. They exploited and violated our women, and demoralized and emasculated our men. They tore our families apart.

Slavery's social impact is clear: poor neighborhoods, inferior schools, lower salaries and wages, limited expectations, diminished hope. What's not so clear is how events that occurred hundreds of years ago could affect our thinking and behavior today. As coauthors Brenda Richardson and the noted psychologist Brenda Wade explain, we can't look at our lives in a vacuum:

[M]any of us go to work each day dressed in our Masters of the Universe suits. We aren't wearing rags that may be stripped from our breasts by a slaveholder

who parades us and our children on an auction block. Yet our unknown great-grandparents' shame lives on in our collective memory. Our history didn't just happen to a group of anonymous people. These people were our ancestors, and in many respects, they are a part of us.[30]

Our ancestors had to learn how to cope in order to survive the raw brutality and utter misery of slavery. Many of their coping strategies obviously served them well, because we're still here. But in return, they paid an enormous psychological price. And today, we're paying interest. To survive, our ancestors learned to act complacent and submissive, in a sense putting on a mask to navigate life. In fact, when defending or talking about sexual attacks by masters or other Whites could lead to punishment such as lashings, sale, or even death, the silence of Black women became a sign of strength and a determination not to allow such experiences to dominate the mind, Wyatt writes. Black women learned to "maintain a certain dignity, a kind of calm resignation, when possible."[31] That lesson was passed from one generation to the next and is still prevalent in many Black families today.

One price they paid, Wyatt writes, was "splitting," or dissociation, a way of thinking that put emotional distance between themselves and the abuse, and memories of the abuse. For example, many survivors talk of "leaving" their bodies, viewing the experience of abuse as if watching from a corner of the room. Or some simply "forget" the experiences altogether. Dissociation made it easier to separate feelings from behaviors, but as experts know today, in spite of our mental efforts to make them go away, such traumas can still surface as sleeplessness, flashbacks, and fears of impending doom.[32] (I will explore dissociation further in Chapter 4: "'Getting It Out' and Healing.")

These coping behaviors were and are quite common among abuse victims, and can persist through generations. "A mother who herself was abused or devalued is not able to protect her child," Wade explains, noting that the mother's behavior is learned. "We are products of what we learn from home. Whatever this generation didn't complete, the next is due to repeat, even if it skips a generation."

Let's look through the prism of our past to get a better sense of the thinking and behaviors we've inherited that allow abuse to occur and continue. Here are some common themes. See if any are familiar.

- **Our bodies are not our own.** Comedians joke, "I brought you into this world—I can take you out!" and we laugh, remembering the terror that our parents' words instilled in us. But many of us believed those kinds of messages. How often were you instructed to "Go on, give your Uncle Junebug a kiss," even when you said you didn't want to? For that matter, you may have even been spanked or punished for disrespecting an adult. When parents force a child to give in to an adult's wishes, the child gets the message that she has no say in what happens to her body and that the adult's needs for affection outweigh her own need for comfort and security. One root of this message is that as enslaved people, we did not control our own bodies. We were a commodity. Anything could be done to us, anytime. And for generations we had little protection or recourse under the law. Many of us are only now becoming comfortable challenging the old norms, by banning spanking, allowing children to be seen and heard, and encouraging them to "talk back" to those in authority if they feel they have good reason to do so.

- **Blacks are hypersexual.** Our ancestors were purchased and sold because of their ability to work *and* breed. After 1807, when the foreign slave trade was abolished, slaveholders looked to the Black women they already had to produce more property.[33] Black men were treated as studs, compared to stallions or bulls, while the women had to bear the seed of the slave master or whichever Black male he sent her way. Few Black women knew of privacy or decorum in the presence of White men. Their bodies were often exposed and even handled at auction, according to historian Deborah Gray White. They often worked in threadbare clothing, and they were stripped for whippings. White men came to equate this exposure and access with sensuality and promiscuity, especially compared with White women, whom they held up as proper and virtuous.[34] Thus, the stereotypes that we can have sex anytime, anywhere, with anybody, and, as Wyatt writes, that we are sexually available for a price. Generations later, we fear these stereotypes so much that we don't talk about sex with our children, and we can't talk about it among adults. Still, we strive to raise "good girls" who keep their skirts down and their knees together, but who are oblivious to what constitutes appropriate sexual behavior. And we often look the other way when abuse happens, not wanting to perpetuate the myths.

- **Black women can tolerate suffering.** From systematic rape at the hands of their masters to abandonment by their own mates, Black women have for generations worn the title of the noble victim. Other races take notice of our "strength."[35] But for many of us, what people perceive as strength is simply the mask we've been wearing since the days of slavery. If we've grown up watching our mothers wear that mask, we've learned to do the same thing. Problem is, as experts say, the thinking—our thinking—becomes that if we can handle suffering, we can handle sexual abuse. And if we think abuse is our burden to bear, we won't blame our abusers.

- **Race matters.** In 1991, a nation tuned in to C-SPAN to watch a Black female law professor named Anita Hill reluctantly testify to fifteen White male Senate Judiciary Committee members that her former boss, Supreme Court nominee Clarence Thomas, had sexually harassed her while she had worked for him at the Equal Employment Opportunity Commission. It was her word against his; he cried foul, speaking of a "high-tech lynching for uppity Blacks," and was ultimately confirmed by the Senate, 52–48. That year we also met Desiree Washington, a Miss Black America Pageant contestant, who accused the heavyweight boxing champion Mike Tyson of rape. Tyson, with a history of attacks against women, was convicted and sentenced to ten years for the crime. When he emerged from prison, many Blacks—from leaders to regular folk—warmly embraced and rallied around him. Washington's name still brings a skeptical response: "That child had no business in his hotel room at all hours of the night." Both women were roundly castigated as turncoats for breaking Black ranks and bringing yet another brother down. The issue of the men's guilt or innocence became secondary. When Black women writers like Ntozake Shange (*For Colored Girls Who Have Considered Suicide, When the Rainbow Is Enuf*), Alice Walker (*The Color Purple*), Toni Morrison (*The Bluest Eye*), and Michele Wallace (*Black Macho and the Myth of the Superwoman*) examined issues of sexual abuse within our families and our community, they too were criticized for "airing our laundry" and "Black-male bashing." The message is clear: As long as we keep silent about sexual abuse, we will continue to sacrifice those who have been victimized for the sake of protecting the race.

- **We are family.** From 1619 to 1865, when our family members were split up and sold away in slavery, others would take in children and the elderly. Today we continue this practice, which is rooted in African tradition, extending the family umbrella beyond our immediate clan to cousins, grands, and others with and without blood ties. This practice of "doubling up" has helped us stay together in spite of adversity.[36] But if we're not careful, we leave our children vulnerable to a relative or family friend to whom we've given access, either by a room or a key, or an unspoken acknowledgment that he or she is one of us. Not everybody who comes under your umbrella of family can live up to the family trust. Not everybody deserves a chance to try.

- **One for all.** Like Darlene, many survivors of abuse feel they must keep quiet for the good of the family. As one sister told me: "I've decided to heal without dragging my family into this." This sense of sacrifice stems from our ancestors' practice of putting family first. As family therapist Nancy Boyd-Franklin writes, "The emphasis in African culture was on the survival of the tribe rather than the individual, the nuclear family or even the extended family."[37] This practice certainly has served us well as a group, but it can be devastating to the survivor who needs to be heard but feels that nobody in her family will listen. A disclosure of abuse forces the family to put the individual first. Many who've been abused end up estranged from their families because they disagree with the "one for all" response to their pain.

- **Ain't nobody's business.** For generations, many of our lives have been pried open, on display, and vulnerable to the dictates of authoritative figures who could use our own information against us. Slave masters. Welfare workers. Social workers. Prosecutors. Judges. Police and parole officers. Even doctors and employers. Among the poor, there is a special sense of powerlessness and rage, writes Boyd-Franklin:

  > To be Black and poor is to live in fear. . . . In many Black inner-city neighborhoods, there are many Black families who are struggling to survive and who feel that they have no protection. Experience has taught them not to trust the police or the courts to deliver justice. Thus they avoid these systems at all costs.[38]

Many of us are wary of exposing sensitive issues to those we don't know or historically have not helped us. Acknowledging abuse exposes us at a most vulnerable point: A crime has been committed and the family is in crisis. Many survivors speak of their mothers' hushed conversations with other adults, trying to "take care of our own" with no professional help. What often happens is that because of fear, ignorance, or denial, nothing gets done. Family members move on with their lives, the abuser is never challenged and in fact still has access to children. And the survivor is left bitter, alone, and with no support.

- **We're too busy for healing.** Our enslaved ancestors spent their days and lives working, tending to others. Emancipation came and went, and most of them found they were still struggling to meet basic needs. For many, life meant labor—sunup to sundown—and no time for self or family. Lynchings left our people terrorized, poverty kept us hungry, and racism kept us fighting. Our biggest job was survival—to keep on keepin' on. And that pushed emotional and psychological healing far down on the to-do list. Sadly, nearly 150 years after emancipation, our priorities are still the same. Many of us don't talk about our emotional and psychological challenges; we simply weren't reared to do that.

We can make a conscious effort to stop this cycle of negative messages and behaviors. But first we need to understand how they affect our lives today. The following chapters will show how families can embrace the lesson that Darlene is slowly learning. Even as she works through her own issues, Darlene has offered to take in one of her nieces while the child's father, Darlene's brother, tries to break a crack habit. Darlene refuses to leave another child vulnerable in her family. She's now looking for her own apartment so she can raise her niece on her own. She's received a promotion at her job and is training to run an after-school program. "I feel like I have a purpose now," she says. "I see opportunities ahead."

And as you begin to untangle the remnants of abuse from the life you want to lead, you should see opportunities too.

HELP YOURSELF

Signs of Abuse? Questions to Ask

Many sexual abuse survivors suffer from post-traumatic stress disorder (PTSD), says Maelinda Turner, a social worker with a managed-care company in San Francisco. "PTSD happens as a result of a trauma or an event that caused a tremendous amount of sustained fear or threat to your life," she says. Symptoms include flashbacks, intense distress, recurrent dreams, and difficulty sleeping and concentrating. Survivors may also have an exaggerated fear of others, outbursts of anger, and depression marked by feelings of hopelessness, crying spells, and a withdrawal from the routines of life. Others may suffer from physical illnesses.

"Identifying with these issues does not necessarily mean you were sexually abused, but knowing the symptoms may enable you to acknowledge past abuse and seek help," Turner says. If you answer yes to three or more of the questions in Turner's checklist below, and answer yes to at least one question in the "What Happened?" checklist (page 13), you most likely were abused and should talk with a trained therapist about your feelings. If you have thoughts of harming or killing yourself, seek help from a trained mental health professional immediately. See Resources for contacts and referrals.

1. Is it difficult for you to trust others?
2. Do you feel threatened when people get too close to you (emotionally and physically)?
3. Do you always feel older than the people around you?
4. Do you have little or no memory of your childhood?
5. Do you have problems with sustaining a love relationship?
6. Do you find unavailable men more attractive than the available ones?
7. Do you have trouble establishing and maintaining boundaries, such as saying no to others?

8. Do you have a number of different sexual partners at a time?
9. Are you obsessed with love relationships?
10. Do you feel disconnected from your body?
11. Do you feel that you are secretive or wearing a mask all the time?
12. Do you feel dirty or ashamed?
13. Do you feel different from other people, as if there is something bad about you?
14. Do you feel like a victim?
15. Do you have persistent feelings of low self-esteem or self-hatred?
16. Do you have a hard time taking care of yourself (for instance, getting enough rest, eating properly, grooming)?
17. Do you feel unable to defend and protect yourself?
18. Do you use work or doing good deeds for others as a way to feel good enough and to compensate for low self-esteem?
19. Are you prone to depression or anxiety attacks?
20. Do you expect people to harm or abuse you?
21. Do you engage in risky sexual behaviors (for instance, with strangers) to make yourself feel wanted or loved?
22. Do you believe that you are good only for sex?
23. When making love, do you feel such fear or anxiety in your body that you desire to be somewhere else?
24. Do you feel that you have to control everything about lovemaking to enjoy it?

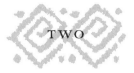

TWO

Overcoming Fear and Shame

There's a mind-body-soul connection. If emotions aren't released,
they hide in the body as disease.

—Social worker MAELINDA TURNER

S O MANY SURVIVORS SUFFER SILENTLY FOR SO MANY REASONS.
As children, we may think that abuse happens to everybody, or that we
deserve what we get. We may feel no one will listen. Or we may not know
the words to describe what happened. Some survivors may not even
remember the sexual abuse, perhaps because it occurred when they were
very young, or because they dissociated, or pushed those painful memories
out of their consciousness. But whether they remember or not, they still
experience the effects. That may explain a feeling of "sleepwalking" through
their days, being alive but not truly living, compressing emotions so they
won't feel pain.

As we grow older and the abuse becomes more distant, other reasons to
keep quiet conveniently crop up. Among them are a lack of time to put healing first; lack of money to pay for counseling; obligations to family, work,
and church; and, as Diane Lewis, who runs a support group for survivors,
puts it: "finding a like-minded and culturally relevant means of intervention
and empowerment." But before we can consider whether our therapist is the
right fit or whether we can fit him or her in our schedule, most of us have to
face two common enemies in conquering sexual abuse: fear and shame.

FACING OUR FEARS

Fear can be overwhelming. It can rule our lives and the lives of others in the family who might be aware of the abuse. Fear keeps us quiet and even makes us resolve to forget that we have been violated. It diminishes us, makes us timid, makes us doubt ourselves and our place in this world. There's the fear of what people will think and what they'll say. There's the fear of retaliation. The fear that you won't be believed. The fear that you'll jeopardize existing relationships. The fear that somebody will go to jail. That somebody will be hurt or die. The fear that you'll be alone. And the fear that you actually invited the abuse. There's the fear that things will never be the same.

Most fears stem from what David Finkelhor, a prolific researcher on sexual abuse, describes as the four major ways in which abuse causes lifelong problems for survivors:[1]

- **Traumatic sexualization.** Distress, confusion, and pain from an inappropriate sexual experience; could lead to obsessions or fears about sex
- **Stigmatization.** Guilt, shame, and self-blame; could lead survivors to feel bad about themselves and hurt themselves
- **Betrayal.** Loss of trust and grief over loss of the relationship, especially when the abuser is related; could lead to difficulty trusting others
- **Powerlessness.** Inability to stop the abuse; could lead to passivity, lashing out, or controlling behavior

When combined with cultural expectations and our notions about our roles as children and women, our problems can keep us from understanding that we've been abused, or keep us from admitting the horror of what really happened. Here's how fears led some women to describe their experiences:

- "But he didn't enter me, he only touched me." (minimizing)
- "It happened so long ago. It's over now." (dismissing)
- "I thought that's what all fathers did to their daughters." (rationalizing)
- "He was drunk. He didn't know what he was doing." (rationalizing)
- "I was sixteen. I felt I should have known better." (self-blame)

GUILT AND SHAME

Many survivors say that guilt and embarrassment play a major role in keeping them quiet. But most often the feelings they are describing are rooted in shame. We need to understand the differences among these emotions and the corrosive nature of shame. We may feel guilty or embarrassed because of something said or done, but we can make that feeling go away by paying a price, be it an apology or some more severe form of restitution, like a term in prison. Shame, however, stems from within. Shame is what we feel not because of what we've done but because of who we are. And as Traci West writes, "because shame has a psychic identity, it can readily emerge with the social stigmas based on race and gender that are usually already at work on Black women's psyches."[3]

Fast Fact

African-American women are less likely than White women to involve police in cases of child sexual abuse.[2]

So when the guilt and embarrassment of sexual abuse are combined with the message that Black women can't control their sexual behavior, for example, it becomes internalized as shame: for being female, for being Black, for *being*. For some survivors of sexual abuse, that shameful feeling is amplified by the emotional abuse of ridiculing and insulting comments by family members. I asked Lori, a Detroit hairstylist who was raped repeatedly by her father starting at age twelve, to tell me how her family might describe her. Her response: "Bitch, evil, and ugly. My sister had long, wavy hair. I had short, kinky hair. Everybody would tell me how ugly I was. And I was evil all the time—always in a mood."

When shame consumes us, it seems there's no price we can pay to make it go away. We don't blame deeds or actions; we blame ourselves. And so to hide what's at the root of our shame, we hide not only the abuse, but a part of ourselves as well. For many of us, harboring secrets can become a way of life. Kristen, whose older cousin repeatedly forced her to have sex with him from ages nine to twelve, says, "There was a real connection between my not telling about the abuse and withholding other things about my life as well. You become good at hiding because you fear that if you don't, others will be able to just look at you and see the shameful truth of what happened to you."

Consider how shame kept these women quiet, and how it affected their lives:

• When she was eight, Rentha, who once was a sex worker in Dallas, was raped so violently by her uncle that she spent a month in the hospital recovering from internal injuries. The attack left her unable to bear children. Rentha's mother, who was high on crack at the time, never asked who had hurt her. Nobody ever explained to the child what had happened to her. So Rentha, who's now twenty-six, explained it to herself this way: "I knew it was something awful, and I knew it wasn't supposed to happen. I thought it was because I had put on my mother's nightgown, or because I rolled my eyes at him that day. And so, when no one said anything I thought, *maybe he punished me because I was bad*." After years of living on the streets, alcohol abuse, and suicide attempts, Rentha found hope through spiritual and psychological counseling. "It's been a struggle," she says. "I put my body through so much. I tormented myself so much because I hated myself for what somebody else had done to me. I'll never do that again. I'll never let anyone make me feel like I'm nothing." But to her, healing has not come so easily. She married a man who loves her dearly, but left him after a few months and headed for the Midwest. She says her husband, Tyrese, deserves better. "I still don't feel I'm good enough." When we last spoke, she was seeing a therapist again, working on feeling good enough for herself first.

• Connie, a forty-one-year-old quiet, reserved sister in Washington, D.C., grew up with her rambunctious older sister under the glare of a strict, controlling mother. They didn't talk much, but when they did, Connie felt her mother's pressure to make up for her sister's ways: "I was considered the good one, the smart one," says the hospital administrator. "People make you feel perfect. They say, 'She's going to go places.'" And Connie played along, becoming a perfectionist. But she found herself hiding from the expectations and attention. "For years my mother would always ask me, 'Why do you have your head down?'" she says. "I always thought my head was up. But to look back on pictures, from ten till about eighteen, it was down." Connie was hiding in shame. It had started when she was ten. A seventeen-year-old friend of the family would catch her alone and kiss and grope her breasts. That feeling of shame continued when the man who ran the corner laundry would feel her up as she dropped off the dry cleaning. Connie knows why she never told her mother about the teenager or the laundry man: She blamed herself for falling short of her mother's expectations. "As a child of somebody who wants things to be so perfect, you don't want to tarnish that image," she says. When she was about sixteen, her mother's boyfriend began to call and ask to see her at home while her mother was at work, and he would slip money under her bedroom door. Connie took the money but never saw him outside of her mother's presence, she says, and she knew there was a sexual nature to his overtures. She kept that from her mother, too. "At one point I said to myself that I didn't want to hurt her feelings," she says. Then she acknowledges the shame she felt for trying to take her mother's man: "Now I think, 'Hmm, maybe I didn't because here was this young little thing and this forty-year-old woman. And she would have felt like I was her competition.'" Connie grew up with few friends because "I didn't want to develop relationships that would allow people to get close," she says. And nobody seemed compatible. "I guess because of all those secrets I needed to try to figure out who I was, because on the outside I was totally different from what was going on inside."

Shame can work against you because you learn that it doesn't matter—that *you* don't matter, says author Brenda Richardson. So you act out. Rentha did so by abusing alcohol, sleeping with men for money, and trying to end her life. Darlene in Chapter 1 did so by leaving home, staying out at all hours, cutting herself. Connie's shame turned inward, and she shielded herself and her secrets from the intimacy of friendship. Each of these women was abused in a different way, and each, in trying to cope in silence, developed mental and behavioral problems that are common among survivors.

Most experts agree that the degree of damage depends not simply on the type of abuse, but on a number of factors involved in the experience. In their book *Breaking Free: A Self-Help Guide for Adults Who Were Sexually Abused as Children,* Carolyn Ainscough and Kay Toon note some of the many factors, including:[4]

- Who the abuser was
- How old the child was
- What took place
- What was said
- How long the abuse went on

- How the child felt and how she interpreted what was happening
- Whether the child was otherwise happy and supported
- How other people reacted to the disclosure or discovery of the abuse

But no matter how severe the damage, eventually the fears must be faced, the shame overcome. The secrets must be dealt with, because the silence that helps us cope in the beginning can lead to mental and physical dysfunction. In general, here are the most common psychological, emotional, and behavioral effects of abuse:[5]

- Depression
- Aggression
- Anxiety
- Delinquency
- Bullying
- Emotional clinging
- Anger
- Flashbacks/intrusion of thoughts
- Feelings of detachment or estrangement from others
- Hostility
- Thoughts of suicide
- Self-destructive behavior
- Concentration and memory problems
- Sleep problems
- Learning difficulties
- Lack of involvement with outside world
- Hyperactivity
- Withdrawal
- Feelings of isolation and stigma
- Poor self-esteem
- Difficulty trusting others
- Eating disorders
- Problems with interpersonal relationships (particularly male-female)
- Substance abuse
- Phobias
- Post-traumatic stress disorder
- Multiple-personality disorder
- Tendency to being revictimized
- Lack of self-confidence
- Nervousness
- Feeling like a victim
- Feeling dirty
- Blackouts
- No interest in sex
- Fear of sex
- Feeling unable to say no to sex
- Avoiding specific sexual activities
- Confusion about sexual orientation
- Inability to love or show affection to children
- Criminal involvement
- Need to be in control

BODILY HARM

Because sexual abuse is a violation of the body, of course obvious physical injury can occur, such as internal and external cuts, bruises, and broken bones. In many cases, however, abuse leaves no physical scars. The lack of obvious signs often makes it difficult for survivors to label their experience as abuse. But the psychological and emotional scars that abuse inflicts can also lead to physical problems, if not immediately, then later in life.

"There's a mind-body-soul connection," says Maelinda Turner, the San Francisco social worker. Turner, who also has a degree in divinity, cites some of the many physical illnesses—obesity, hypertension, sexual dysfunction, and reproductive problems—that can stem from traumatic experiences like sexual abuse and the silence that surrounds it. "It may sound New Agey," Turner says, "but if emotions aren't released, they hide in the body as disease. The emotion sits there, and stress and your lifestyle feed that disease."

Lori, the sister from Detroit who recently sought help for severe depression, tells of the unhealthy cycle that she's been in: "I feel like I have an old body compared to my mind. I'm the biggest I've ever been. Stressed out. Just out of control." That stress would lead Lori to overeat and ignore her health, and she'd gain still more weight and become even more depressed. Now, she says, "I'm getting control over what I eat, taking control over how I work and when I work. And my personal life. For the longest time, I felt I had no control." With the help of her therapist, whom friends urged her to see, Lori made the connection between her father's abuse and her feeling out of control. "When I would say no, bad things would happen to me," she says. "I would get beat. I would get punished. It was better not to say no. I was tired of being hurt all the time."

On the following pages, you will meet three sisters who have vastly different stories, but at the root of each is childhood sexual abuse, silence, and the fears and shame that surround it. Each woman shares how the abuse and silence have affected her life, and how she has responded. I've asked experts to review their experiences and explain the emotional and psychological dynamics at play and how the women can move forward. At the end of the chapter you will find exercises to begin a discussion on abuse, even within yourself, and to help draw others out if you suspect they've been abused.

STEPHANIE'S STORY: DANGEROUS GAMES

"When Mama was away, my father would put us on his lap and feel us up," says Stephanie, the second of three sisters from a rural midwestern town. "He'd call us into his room one at a time. He would start with a hug or a tickle, and all of a sudden he would be touching my breasts. We all knew what was happening. My sisters and I had this code. We'd say, 'Okay, in five minutes, you've got to come and get me.'"

It is not often that Stephanie, a thirty-two-year-old artist, makes her way from her East Coast home back to the home where she grew up. It reminds her of the "games" the girls had to play with their father. Throughout the girls' childhood, their father would call on the oldest sister most often. Today that sister escapes the pain of those memories through the use of illegal drugs and alcohol. Stephanie's youngest sister struggles with overeating.

On the surface, Stephanie, who is single, seems highly functional compared with her sisters. She is full of energy, has a host of friends, jammed workweeks and weekends packed with theater dates, parties, and book-club gatherings. You will rarely find her waiting around for something to happen; she goes out and creates the action. Since she left the family home for college, she has never looked back.

Turner, the San Francisco social worker, sees patterns typical of sexual abuse victims in Stephanie and her sisters. "You can always find ways to avoid the pain by escaping it," she explains. "Work, drugs, food. You can be successful and smart and busy, but eventually it's going to sneak up on you. At some point you need to slow down and deal with what happened and how it has affected your life."

When I ask Stephanie how she feels about what her father did to her and her sisters, and about the years of silence that followed, she seems surprised. She's never thought much about it, she says, adding, "What's done is done." But a moment later, she changes course. "Things have been building up over the last couple of years," she admits. "I'm at the point where I hate when my father even answers the phone. Yet when I do go home, I don't want him to know that I feel uncomfortable. He's this old man and he does love me. It's all bizarre."

Stephanie believes the abuse she suffered at her father's hands is to blame for her struggle to become truly intimate with men. "For a long time, I didn't like to be touched," she says. "It made me feel kind of helpless." Her sisters, too, have had trouble sustaining intimate relationships. Both have never married, but each has a child.

"The great wound of sexual abuse," Turner explains, "is that it leads you to believe that you are not worthy to celebrate the gifts of the power of your sexuality without fear, question, or judgment." I ask Stephanie if she and her sisters have ever considered talking with a professional. "I don't know," she says with a shrug. "I feel like you're supposed to just go on with your life."

Turner stresses that unless their father gets help, the sisters must know that as long as their children are around him, they too will be in danger. That fear is quite real. A few years ago, one sister suspected their father had begun to abuse her six-year-old son. Her fear for her son led her to confront her father about the abuse she and her sisters had suffered. As the secret came tumbling out, her mother reacted with disbelief. "You all must have done something," she said lamely, not knowing how else to respond. The father insisted that nothing had happened with the sisters or the grandson, and the mother let the issue drop. Stephanie's sister, dismayed by her parents' denial and feeling the need to protect her son, now steers clear of her parents' home.

Talking about sex makes many of us uncomfortable, and discussing sexual abuse is even more difficult. People don't know what to say, or they just want it to go away. Well-meaning parents may never again bring up the subject after confronting an abuser, or—not wanting to believe that Daddy or Cousin Harold could do such a thing—may tell a child that perhaps she misunderstood. Either response causes "secondary injuries," as experts describe a lack of proper support. Such injuries leave the child struggling alone to deal with the abuse, along with its residual feelings of shame and self-doubt.

That episode was the first and last time Stephanie and her sisters ever openly discussed the abuse with their parents. Turner believes that the entire family will need to go into therapy if healing is to occur. She feels that Stephanie might be the person in her family who could initiate that—if she starts by helping herself. "Often, one person in the family can take the lead," Turner says. "Stephanie seems to have the clearest sense of who she is and how [the abuse] has shaped her. She also has a strong support system of friends. She could talk to her sisters. It's clear from their experience that they have a caring, protective relationship."

But while healing for the family may require a team effort, Stephanie's first obligation is to herself. She can encourage her family to go into counseling, but as many survivors eventually realize, she needs to accept that she may have to move on without them. Turner acknowledges that it is unlikely that Stephanie's parents will ever move past their denial enough to enter therapy. Mothers who can't acknowledge their daughters' abuse have often been abused themselves, she reflects. Until they can deal with their own demons, they can't begin to help their daughters. "It's like a cancer," Turner says. "If your grandmother had it and your mother had it, you're susceptible."

As for her father, Stephanie is resigned. "People are who they are," she says. "Rather than have him live out his last days being miserable, I've made a conscious decision to make him feel comfortable." A soft sigh escapes her as she adds: "That just leaves me waiting until he dies."

EVELYN'S STORY: SEX FOR SALE

Evelyn's eyes could pass for fifty, though she is only thirty-eight. She grew up in a comfortable home in New York City with her parents, sister, and two brothers. When she was ten, her brother's teenage friend began to creep up to her bedroom to fondle her. He'd give her candy to keep her silent. Evelyn finally threatened to tell only when he pressured her to "let him put his thing in me." After that, he left her alone. In junior high, she fell into a clique of girls who regularly visited the principal's office. "We let him feel us up, and he gave us money and good grades," she says. The principal was fired when one of the girls became pregnant and told. No one else in the clique breathed a word.

At sixteen, Evelyn befriended a man who owned a neighborhood store. He invited her into the basement for drugs and sex. Not long after, she got pregnant by him and dropped out of school to have the child. She was in the ninth grade and could barely read. "I was always used to a man taking care of me," she says. "I always wanted nice things." At eighteen she met Tommy, who fed her crack habit and then beat her. Desperate to escape him, Evelyn left her baby with her mother and took off on her own. Soon, she was selling her body to buy crack. "It didn't matter what they did to me," she says of the countless tricks she turned. "I just wanted my money."

Gail Wyatt, the expert on Black women and sexuality, observes that by the time she was a teenager, Evelyn had been conditioned to see herself as a sexual object and sex as a means to an end. Evelyn's case is extreme, Wyatt notes, but in all sexual relationships it's important to ask, "Is my body just being used to get me something?"

Evelyn quickly spiraled into a routine of sex, violence, and drugs that consumed two decades of her life and drained every ounce of her self-worth. In crack houses, she would emerge from her haze naked and bruised, knowing she had been raped. "I was too afraid to go to the cops," she says. "Why would they believe me? I wanted to die. I remember asking God why I wasn't dying." She was too ashamed to tell her family that she needed help. "I didn't want them to see me; I didn't want to disgrace them," she says.

Her unwillingness to reveal to her family her earliest incidents of abuse—first by her brother's friend, then by the principal, and later by the store owner—may have played a role in Evelyn's later history of abusive sexual encounters. As Wyatt observes, the dynamics within a family are frequently at the root of our silence around issues of sex and sexuality. "Often the abuse victim is a needy person whose family has not responded to that," Wyatt explains. "The decision not to tell says a lot about whom they trust, their sense of loneliness and isolation. Sometimes there's an emotional distance within the family. It's difficult to talk about sex if you're not talking about other things in general. And if you talk to perpetrators, they'll tell you they can sense vulnerable, needy kids."

Evelyn, still vulnerable and needy as an adult, eventually entered an upstate drug treatment program, where her pattern continued: She had sex for money with men on staff. She got caught and kicked out, and headed back to the streets. "I was out of control," she remembers. "I'd sleep on rooftops and in hallways. I'd wake up next to men and not know who they were or how I got there." In all, she had four children, two of them by tricks. They all live with her mother. Evelyn was arrested a few times, and the last time they found drugs on her. She landed in Project Greenhope, a Manhattan alternative-to-incarceration rehabilitation and drug treatment center for women. When I meet her eight months later, she's clean, mercifully AIDS-free and, through counseling, is beginning to understand the roles that sexual abuse and silence have played in her life. When she left the treatment center, she was on her own for the first time, and with $117 a month in welfare, she was looking for a job and a home. "I'm learning to love myself, but I'm scared to death," she admits. "I've never paid a bill in my life."

While Wyatt applauds Evelyn's efforts to turn her life around, she cautions that Evelyn will need long-term psychotherapy to get to the root of the abuse and silence that have so derailed her life. And Evelyn, who was conditioned to give her own power away, needs to learn about her own power over her body. Wyatt says Evelyn also needs to develop strong relationships with positive women, perhaps other graduates of her treatment center, and she must avoid the temptations of old friends and old habits. She encourages Evelyn to avoid sexual relationships altogether until she can get in touch with her own sexuality. "Until now she's been operating on someone else's agenda," Wyatt says. "This is not just about sex; this is her whole life."

Since our interview, Evelyn has disappeared, and her counselors don't know whether her recovery has continued.

KIM'S STORY: LONGING FOR LOVE

Behind Kim's fiery spirit and quick wit is a wounded, still-grieving young woman. She's overweight, but, she says, "I have too many other things to work on" to worry about dropping pounds. She's single and often lonely, even when she was with her most recent boyfriend for seven years. Before him, by her own account, she had a string of mostly empty sexual relationships, forty in all. "I used to confuse sex with love," she says. She still finds it difficult to believe that a man could want more than sex from her. "I'm always afraid that people will leave if they see the real me."

Kim can identify exactly when these feelings of worthlessness began. Her stepfather started fondling her during bath time when she was about seven, and by the time she was eleven, he had graduated to intercourse. Looking back, Kim can see that he was priming her for sex all along. "I went through several stages, from crying to just giving in to fighting to get him away from me," says the thirty-four-year-old. She felt she had no choice but to remain silent: Her stepfather had warned that if she told her mother, a prominent southern political and church activist, he would kill them both. To prove his point, he'd often sharpen his knives and clean his gun in front of Kim.

And so, while Mom was out saving the world, Kim endured routine rapes by the man who was supposed to be taking care of her, beatings whenever she threatened to tell, and a pregnancy and horrifying miscarriage that she suffered through alone at age sixteen. "I knew my stepfather was the father," she wrote in a journal of her experiences, "and just like everything else he had done to me, I could not tell anyone about it."

When Kim was nineteen, her stepfather pressed one time too many for sex. She resisted and he slapped her, and in her anger she found the courage to tell her mother. Kim's mother responded by accusing her of seducing her stepfather and ordering her out of the house. She lived with friends and family for a while before moving out on her own. Many years later, she would learn that her mother had herself been sexually abused by a relative. Through therapy she would come to understand that her mother, wounded herself, had no idea how to comfort or support her daughter. At the time, though, Kim was devastated.

"Sometimes I think I shouldn't have said anything," Kim says through tears. "I paid a price for telling: I had to change my life. I had never lived anywhere else. I had no degree, no job, no skills. I didn't have anybody but me. I lost a good part of my life." She tries to describe the physical and psychological impact of her past: "It's why I constantly have indigestion. Whenever I get afraid, I want to throw up. I'm always waiting for the other shoe to drop, always waiting for something to rock my semblance of being normal."

Dorothy Cunningham, a clinical psychologist with a private practice in New York, explains that Kim's situation was compounded by her mother's denial. "When a parent refuses to accept what's going on, they're often thinking about what it could do to their career and to their family," Cunningham says. "It took a great deal of courage for Kim to say this happened, and the mother left her child to heal herself."

Kim is now working toward her college degree. She's been in therapy for years, though she admits she doesn't go as often as she should. "Sometimes it's just too hard," she says. "Sometimes it makes me so uncomfortable." And yet therapy is crucial to Kim's healing process, Cunningham says. "There's a loss of innocence, a loss of childhood and of family," she explains, and it's important for abuse victims to mourn that loss. Therapy can be a safe place to do that.

Cunningham also sees in Kim a woman who needs to get angry. "People who stay in victim mode never get to the anger point," she says. "They blame themselves; they see themselves as bad and dirty. In some ways that's safer than unleashing the anger that's inside. You need to give yourself permission to be angry. Say: 'I deserve to be listened to, I deserve protection.' When you're a victim, you don't feel like you deserve anything. When you're angry, you're empowered."

One of the most difficult memories for an abuse victim to deal with is the sensation of pleasure that her body may have experienced. Even now, Kim struggles to understand how she could have felt pleasure while being raped. "It was like looking forward to a lover," she says, her voice almost a whisper. "And as much as I looked forward to it, it repulsed me too."

As disturbing as Kim finds this aspect of her abuse, her experience is not uncommon. "It's very difficult for many to accept," Cunningham confirms. "You can be terrified and confused but still have an orgasm. Kim should know that her body did what bodies are supposed to do—it responded to touch. That's how bodies are made. She needs to know that she's not a perverted soul."

Ten years ago, after Kim's stepfather died, she began to reach out to her mother. But their conversations often spiral into accusations and tears. Though she still longs for the nurturing that she feels she missed while growing up, Kim recognizes that she is more likely to get it from supportive friends and family members than from her mother. "She is what she is," Kim sums up, "but I still love her. And I know I'm going to be okay."

BREAKING THE SILENCE

Though every case of sexual abuse is different, some common therapeutic themes emerge. We need to speak out about our experience, because only in doing so will we get rid of the burden of secrecy and begin to move our lives forward. We must recognize that the simple act of telling about assault is a form of resistance, because doing so makes it "possible for the crime to be known and remembered," as Traci West writes.[6]

We need to work on the effects of abuse by understanding the role of power in our relationships, and by holding abusers accountable for their actions. *It doesn't matter what the child does; abuse is the fault of the abuser.* So we must forgive ourselves to release the shame, and treat ourselves gently as we come to terms with our past.

We also need to know that the treatment we seek will take time. "It is difficult to know how long," Maelinda Turner says of the healing process. "You can't mark progress or breakthroughs, but you can look back in six months or a year and know that you're in a different place. On the other hand, you can have a breakthrough with as little as a word that the therapist says." For Evelyn and Kim, talk therapy helped them learn and articulate how the abuse shaped their lives, powerful steps toward healing. Stephanie, who seems resigned to keeping her father's abuse of her and her sisters in the past, can't allow herself to be introspective and doesn't see talk therapy as very useful. But she may find solace with another kind of therapy, like art or dance. Chapter 4 ("'Getting It Out' and Healing") explores these and other holistic approaches, like writing and music.

So what prompts a survivor to end the silence, to go beyond the fear and shame to the help on the other side? Evelyn was forced to confront her fears or run the risk of relapse and prison. Connie realized she avoided nurturing friendships. Kim was "tired of being sick and alone and tired." Lori was saved by a girlfriend, who, fearing that Lori would hurt herself, took her to see a therapist. When the burden becomes too much to bear, it is released. How that burden is received can be critical to a survivor's recovery. And that's why family members are so important to the healing process. I will explore the role of family in Chapter 3.

HELP YOURSELF

Understanding Roots of Silence

These two exercises will help you break the silence, even if it's within yourself, and help you assist someone you suspect has been abused. The first exercise is adapted from *Breaking Free: A Self-Help Guide for Adults Who Were Sexually Abused as Children.*[7]

1. Look at the list of reasons why children don't tell that they are being abused. Check any that applied to you. See if you can think of others.

Why children don't tell

No one to tell
Parents dead, ill, absent
Parents involved in abuse
No trustworthy adult around
No opportunity to talk alone with a trusted adult
Caregivers do not listen or are unresponsive
Frightened of parents
Parents discourage talk about sex
No friends

No way to say it
The child is too young to talk
The child doesn't know how to describe what is happening
The child is too embarrassed and ashamed to say

Fears about the consequences of telling
• **Threats from the abuser**

No one will believe
The child will be put into a home
The child will not see her mother/caretaker again
The family will be split up
Affection and love will be withdrawn
Family and friends will reject the child
No one will want to marry her
Threatened or actual physical violence to the child, family, or pets
The abuser will kill himself or be put in prison

• **Fears concerning others' reactions**
No one will believe the child
Mother will feel guilty
Family will be hurt
Mother will reject the child
Other people will think child is to blame
Other people will think the child is dirty, contaminated, or disgusting
The child will be rejected and the abuser supported

• **Fears for the abuser**
He will be hurt and rejected
He will be put in prison
He will get beaten up
He will kill himself

• **Fears that telling won't help**
Nothing will change
No one can stop it
Events will get out of control
Fear of the unknown
It might get worse
The abuser is too powerful for anyone to stop

• **Confused feelings and thoughts**
Guilt, self-blame, shame, embarrassment
Uncertainty: Is it really happening? Is it wrong?
Thinking the abuse is normal
Not understanding what is happening
Believing she is the only one this has ever happened to

Feeling dirty, contaminated, polluted
Trapped by the secrecy
Feeling she is being punished and deserves it
Hoping the abuse won't happen again
Blocking off all memories of the abuse
Feeling sorry for the abuser
Not wanting to betray the abuser by telling
Feeling it's her fault because she took candy, money, toys, or other
    rewards from the abuser
Enjoying the sexual stimulation
Enjoying the affection, warmth, or closeness

Your additional reasons:

_____

_____

_____

_____

_____

2. In your journal or diary, write your own account of why you didn't tell anyone at the time the abuse was occurring.

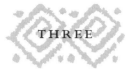

THREE

Family Matters: Moving Beyond Denial

I didn't take it serious enough.

—ALLEN, who acknowledged his thirty-five-year-old daughter's abuse,
more than twenty years after she disclosed it

WHEN I WAS A GIRL, IT SEEMED THAT EVERYBODY IN MY FAMILY knew about a certain older cousin, who, whenever he hugged younger female relatives, would manage to withdraw an arm in such a way that a hand would linger long enough to brush a nipple or quickly squeeze a breast or buttock. But nobody would say a word, and so the girls were left to try to outmaneuver this cousin or, if they found themselves in his embrace, squirm their way out before he could get his hands on them. Perhaps no one thought it was serious enough to warrant pulling his coat and standing up for the girls. But that open secret sent a powerful message to the young women kin: their physical safety and comfort were not as important as the sexual urges of a man, and when it came to our menfolk taking advantage of them, they were on their own.

Physical violation is traumatic, but even more devastating is abuse by someone you know, trust, and love.[1] Survivors of child sexual abuse are often doubly traumatized—betrayed first by the abuser and then again by other family members who fail to protect or fail to believe them once they tell.

In its stark, scholarly fashion, *Webster's Collegiate Dictionary* defines *family* as "a group of individuals living under one roof," and also as "a group of persons of common ancestry." In the real world, family encompasses those definitions and so much more: our anchor and foundation, our support, our hope, a source of love and understanding, a force that nurtures, sustains, revitalizes, influences, encourages, accepts, and protects.

For a child who is abused by a family member, all the meanings of family and her foundation for being—her very core—are distorted and damaged. Where is her anchor if her anchor is the source of her pain? Where does she go for protection and understanding if she is blamed for her abuser's actions? Where does she find nurturing and protection if those who are charged to do so ignore her plight? Whom does she turn to? Most often—feeling that she comes last in the family pecking order, or feeling that her problems aren't important, or feeling that she somehow caused the abuse—she turns inward. And, without the support or tools to heal, she is rarely equipped to help herself.

Before we look at flaws in our families that allow abuse to happen, we must remember the context. Our families are no more or less dysfunctional than those of other races or ethnicities. But we cannot overestimate the impact that slavery and systemic racism have on our family dynamics, and how the still-pervasive fear of institutional racism and its agents keeps our families from reporting abuse to the authorities.

Often an underlying reason is that survivors don't feel they *deserve* help and protection, and that feeling, too, has its roots in oppression.

For years social scientists and policy makers characterized many of our families as abnormal: unstable, broken, disadvantaged, deprived. They pointed out direct links to fatherlessness, juvenile delinquency, dependence on the "system," and a drag on public resources.[5] This "deficit view," as family therapist Nancy Boyd-Franklin describes it, perceived the Black family structure as "nonconformist and fundamentally pathological."[6] The media (including but not limited to movies, television, newspapers, and mag-

Fast Facts

- One study showed that Black girls were more often abused than Whites by relatives other than their fathers. Often the offender was an uncle.[2]

- The study also showed that Black women reported "more upset, greater long-term effects, and more negative life experiences" from sexual abuse than White women.[3]

- Incestuous abuse of Blacks was more than three times more likely to be "very severe" (involving oral, anal, or vaginal intercourse) compared with that of Whites, according to the study, and to involve force or physical violence and verbal threats.[4]

azines) often back up the view by presenting Black pathology as if it is our only dimension. And, sadly, many of us have bought into it ourselves.

While many researchers, like Boyd-Franklin, have challenged this deficit view in the last twenty years, the vestiges of bias and lingering stereotypes are still with us and often emerge at the most unfortunate time: when Blacks seek help from White institutions and find little sympathy or understanding.

Anyone who has any doubt about the strength and resilience of Black people should consider where we've come from and what it took for us to get here today. Snatched from our homes and families. Piled into the hulls of ships teeming with disease and waste and agony. Dumped onto the shores of an unfamiliar land, to do the work of mules. Stripped of our languages, our religions, our autonomy, and our memories, beaten into submission, we lived under the most inhumane conditions. Or we died. No other group of people has endured what we did. We exist because our ancestors survived. We are the very reason they survived.

Black Americans are a people of unwavering strength in the face of the most insurmountable challenges: two hundred fifty years of slavery and its post-Reconstruction spawn, Jim Crow. Then modern-day social and economic racism and institutional apathy and brutality. Through perseverance, faith, and fellowship, we're still here. One of the main factors in our survival is the strength of our families and in many cases our extended families. Unfortunately, for so many of us, our strengths have long concealed weaknesses, passed down from one generation to the next, and our survival has come at a price. The psychological toll can be likened to that of a soldier fighting a war. Though the battlefields have changed over the years, we are still in combat. Today, we suffer trauma in our neighborhoods, our workplaces, and our schools. It can be seen in the lack of adequate housing and affordable health care, in chronic unemployment and underemployment, and in waking up each day facing fear.

Many of us are emotionally scarred and numb—unable to love, unable to experience our own feelings, and unable to be open and honest with one another. We've come through the fire, but we got burned. We've got "issues," among them anxiety, addiction, mental and physical illness, economic insecurity, limited opportunities, and an all-too-common sense of hopelessness and despair. Abuse can flourish in a family with issues.

Those family issues are like an Achilles' heel, the weak spot in our collective strength, the blind spot in our collective sight. But when we deal with our dysfunction, acknowledging and working on our weaknesses, our families can be truly strong—wholly strong—and our children valued and protected.

THE RIPPLE EFFECT

Child sexual abuse can affect every member of the family. Children disclose, and adults must respond in one way or another, or else children carry the shameful secret, which will lead to behavioral problems or mental and physical disorders. Eventually, everyone pays a price for the abuse or the secrets. Here are ways in which family members may be affected.

Children

Oftentimes adults know something is up, but they don't recognize abuse as a problem because children tend to tell without "telling." Ellen Bass and Laura Davis suggest in their book *The Courage to Heal:*

> If children don't tell with words, they often tell through behavior. They wet beds. They steal from a parent's wallet. They are terrified to go to sleep, and wake up screaming from nightmares. . . . They don't want to be left alone. They develop asthma. They stop eating. They have trouble in school. They cry hysterically every time [the abuser] comes over. They demonstrate a precocious interest in sex. They act seductively to get things they want. . . . Older children or teenagers act out by disobeying or getting into trouble with authorities. They become depressed, take drugs or engage in self-destructive behavior. They are trying to get someone to pay attention, but the behavior is usually misinterpreted.[7]

Siblings

As children, siblings of survivors often carry the knowledge that a sister or brother is victimized, and live with the fear that they could be next. In Stephanie's case, in which she and her sisters were abused by their father, the three girls developed an elaborate scheme of distractions to interrupt the abuse. In her home, no child was safe, so the children bore the burden of saving one another. They worked to keep the abuse from their mother, and the lie strained their ties with her. Today, Stephanie and her sisters find it difficult to have intimate relationships with men.

In some cases, if a sibling learns about another's abuse, the child may be pushed to choose sides in a battle of family loyalty. A sibling may resent the one who was abused, thinking she sought attention. Or there may be bitterness that one sibling got out of the house and left others to fend for themselves.

Spouses / Partners of Abusers

The partner of an abuser can also be a victim. Her faith in their partnership is destroyed. She is embarrassed and questions her own judgment in choosing a mate. How could she have lived with this person, she wonders, sharing her most intimate self, rearing his children, fighting battles and celebrating victories, to have him not simply cheat on her, but to have sex with a child? If it is her own children who are abused, she feels enormous guilt for not protecting them, and if she, too, is a survivor, she may experience painful memories of her own abuse.

Brenda's husband, Charles, is serving seven to fifteen years in an Ohio medium-security prison for the repeated molestation of Brenda's daughter, Karla, his stepdaughter. Brenda is rare, experts say: When she found out about the abuse, she immediately reported her husband to the authorities. (We will learn more about their story in Chapter 7, "Challenging Abusers.") Not only was she furious that her husband victimized her daughter, but she was also devastated that his actions cost them their relationship. In her journal, after she confronted Charles, Brenda wrote: "I felt like my world had literally crumbled around me. I felt confused, hurt and in disbelief. I thought I'd finally found a decent man with strong family values and ties. One who confessed everlasting commitment and love. There's no more security, nowhere to lay my head on his chest."

Later she shared: "We had a very healthy sex life, and we were very affectionate with each other. And that's one of the things that hurt so much, you know, that he was with me when he was doing these things with my daughter."

Parents of Abusers

In a case of abuse between adolescents or children, parents may find themselves torn between loyalty to a child who is the abuser and loyalty to the survivor. For Ann, a Chicago mother of three, the struggle was even more pronounced, because both the abuser and the survivor were her children. In her role as an office manager, Ann is a skilled problem solver. But this was the biggest challenge of her life. Reluctantly, she remembers the anguish she felt when she learned of her daughter's experience, and how she fought through it to support both her children.

"My youngest daughter, Shauna, was abused by her stepbrother," Ann says. "When she told me, about four years ago, she was in her freshman year in high school. Her grades weren't good. We'd just moved to a more integrated neighborhood, the most diverse she'd ever been in. We were meeting with teachers, and Shauna would come home with racial stories. She was having a terrible, terrible time.

"One day she said she didn't want to go back. I remember I said, 'Oh no, baby, you can't run away from your situation.' And she began sobbing uncontrollably. I called my husband and told him to come home. She seemed to be having a nervous breakdown. At home, we kept asking her, 'What's wrong? You can tell us.'" Now Ann herself begins to cry, "And that's when she just burst out, 'OK! I'll tell you! I was abused by Richard!'" The abuse had happened when Shauna was about three until she was seven, Ann recalls as she wipes away tears. Richard is six years older, so he was nine to thirteen. They have an older sister, Carolyn, "But Shauna and Richard were inseparable," Ann says. "Shauna didn't understand what Richard was doing to her. I think when she got older and became more aware of her body, she understood. At school, she didn't seem to fit in with Black people or White people. She had to find her way in the middle. And I think with her having to reach deep inside herself to find that strength, that she reached and pulled up the pain."

Ann remembers her confusion and the distance that grew between her and her husband, Harold: "Here I was trying to deal with the fact that my only child had been sexually abused by her stepbrother. I didn't know how to relate to Shauna. And Harold, well, he even questioned if she was telling the truth. He even said, 'Well, you know this goes on all the time in other families.' As if we were supposed to accept it. It just put a wedge in everybody's communication."

Fortunately, Carolyn, Shauna's stepsister, stepped in to help, by talking with her sister and mediating between all parties. "She was so supportive of her sister," Ann says. Ann found a support group and a therapist, whom Shauna saw for about six months.

But Ann also remembers the guilt and self-questioning. "I just felt like, 'What kind of parent was I? What was so much more important than protecting her?'" And she struggled to face her stepson. "I hated him. I didn't want to talk to him when I'd see him. I didn't want him in my house. My husband had to confront him."

And when her husband did confront him months later, Richard told the truth. "And he said, 'Dad, I'm so sorry,'" Ann recalls. "And he came and apologized to me, and he cried and cried. And he and Shauna talked. It was amazing seeing my babies acting like adults." Ann says it took about half a year to open her heart to Richard again. "Then, when I saw him, he was my son again. When he apologized, and when I knew Shauna would be OK, I knew I couldn't just cast him out." While Richard atoned for the pain he caused his stepsister and his family, he began using drugs, and, like Ann's husband, did not seek counseling.

Ann's experience is not unusual. Not every member of a family will agree or acknowledge that sexual abuse has occurred, even when it's plain to see.

Extended Family

Other relatives might struggle with guilt by association. Vonetta, who runs a charter school in a small Ohio town, is the sister of Charles, who is in prison for abusing his stepdaughter, Karla. Vonetta can't contain her disappointment and disgust. "He treated her like a woman, but she was just six years old," Vonetta says. "It's so embarrassing. I'd rather him be in prison for drugs. People know him, and I have friends who know him."

She often avoids the truth when some people ask about Charles: "I don't say he's in prison, 'cause then they'll ask why. I say he blew town. And they say, 'He's a sorry father for neglecting his responsibilities.' And I just say, 'Yeah, he made that choice.'"

Mostly she fears that Charles's actions will affect her own professional aspirations. "There was a time when I wanted to be mayor of our town. I felt that I could make a run and make a change, but then I realized that somebody would do a background check. And I would never want that to come out. I think about how that would reflect on me."

In the end, she's managed to support her niece and to begin to support her brother. "I love my brother, you know. I just don't love the act he did."

Having a sexual abuser in the family is not easy to acknowledge or accept. Vonetta and her family are working through some of the tough problems that Charles's crime and punishment have raised among them. But the family is also finding ways to cope and heal. The alternative would have been to ignore Charles's illness and his crime, as well as the pain he was inflicting on his stepdaughter. And with that silent and tacit blessing, all other children who came into contact with him would have been at risk of being abused.

THE SECRETS WE KEEP

Family therapist Nancy Boyd-Franklin writes that there are two kinds of secrets: those that are kept from outsiders but are known by most family members, and those that are kept from other family members. The first type is an open secret, generally known but not discussed. The second is a form of deception. Secrets can live for generations just behind a family's façade. In her therapy work, Boyd-Franklin notes, "It is not unusual to discover that there is awareness on the part of family members that there are secrets or loaded issues that are never discussed."[8] Both types of secrets can devastate relationships and family ties.

Certainly ours aren't the only families that harbor secrets, but because of a host of reasons, including our mistrust of authorities and a desire to support Black men, often in spite of themselves, we are more likely to keep our business "out of the streets" and not seek intervention or professional help. To Boyd-Franklin's list of the most common secrets among our families (informal adoption and true parentage, fatherhood, unwed pregnancy, mental illness, drug abuse, alcoholism, ancestry, skin-color issues), we can certainly add sexual abuse.

Keeping abuse an open secret within the family not only fails the survivor and excuses the abuser's behavior, but also strains relationships within the family and without. In many cases people don't know what to do when they see or hear that one of the clan is an abuser. If they believe it (which family alliances and politics may keep them from doing), they're shocked, disgusted, and embarrassed. Extended-family members thank their lucky stars it wasn't them or their kids. And then they keep it to themselves. This kind of denial—knowing something happened, but not acknowledging it—can devastate a survivor.

The following story gives us a clear idea of how even the most well-meaning parents can create a space in which abuse can happen, and the price that family members pay when they don't acknowledge it. Life is messy and so are folks' recollections. Sometimes stories don't add up, and people disagree on what was said when. Fortunately for this survivor, and for her parents, they've managed to look beyond those details and find a path toward healing.

MAYA'S (AND HER PARENTS') STORY:
CAUGHT IN THE MIDDLE

Maya, the daughter of civil and human rights activists, grew up "in the struggle." The thirty-five-year-old Baltimore artist and activist had a young life of marches, meetings, and demonstrations. "As a child," she says, "I hated the Movement. I would say, 'I just want a normal family.'" Both parents have traveled extensively. Her father did jail time for protests and civil disobedience. Her mother became a local women's and spiritual leader. But in spite of their common sense of activism, Maya's parents were polar opposites when it came to a host of issues, including raising their daughter. They separated shortly before Maya went to kindergarten. In the turbulent trenches of her parents' lives, Maya was left vulnerable, and was abused by her father's stepfather. Her parents played hot potato with her disclosure, until Maya, using their own brand of activism, began to speak out about sexual abuse and forced them to acknowledge her experience and the roles they played in it. Here are their accounts.

MAYA

My parents were in this ideological struggle with me around religion, around other things—so, in many ways, that left me confused and caught in the middle. In hindsight, I know they were struggling over my identity and my mind-set. My mother wanted me to have the best in everything—private schools and all that. My father was opposed to those kinds of things.

My grandmother—my father's mother—played a major role in my upbringing because my parents traveled so much. Gram's house was my house. I had a room and everything. I went to school from there. And I was very, very close to her and to her husband, whom I call my grandfather. She was definitely like a mother. There were times that I wished she *was* my mother.

With my grandfather, I was very much the favorite grandchild. For Christmas and my birthday, he would always give me some huge gift—Barbie and all that kind of stuff. My grandparents married in the '60s. She didn't work outside the house. So she was almost always home.

When I was about ten, one of my dad's brothers became very sick, and Gram was on, around the clock, taking care of her son at the hospital. She was away, physically and emotionally. It was during this time that my grandfather, Poppy, started to fondle me. He would kiss me and force me to kiss him. With his tongue. And he'd do these head trips. Like when my cousins were around, he'd say to me, "Oh, don't you want to kiss me?" And I would say, "No, I don't want to kiss you." And one of the cousins would go, "Oh, I'll kiss you Poppy! I'll kiss you!" But he would kiss the cousin like an adult should kiss a child.

I was starting to develop my breasts and all of that, so, needless to say, it was all very uncomfortable. And it was very intense, because I told my grandmother every single thing but that. So that was the beginning of my keeping secrets.

One night, my grandfather came home from work when we were asleep—he sometimes worked the night shift—and I remember him sitting on the side of my bed and touching my vagina. I remember not being asleep and not knowing what to do, so I just acted like I was asleep and tossed and turned. Eventually, he stopped and left. It was at that point that I told my mother.

I can't really remember how or what I said. But her initial thing was, "Are you sure you weren't dreaming?" And she just kept asking me and asking me to the point where I wasn't sure if it was real. That definitely has had an effect to this day—about not being sure, even though I know something happened.

My mother questioned me—around 1999 to 2000. We went through a lot of stuff. I always blamed her in a way that I never even blamed my father. I blamed her for not rescuing me. One of the reasons I had so much rage toward her was that I thought she only cared about how this would affect her arrangements for a permanent babysitter. Everybody was traveling, so this meant, where was Maya going to stay?

I started lying all the time—about school, about everything. I was setting my parents up against each other, because I knew all their buttons. My mother raised me as a vegetarian; I would lie and say Daddy would give me meat—just constantly set stuff up. I was a terror.

When my dad caught me in another lie, and he was telling me about how he caught me, he said—and I'll never forget this—"And another thing, I talked to Poppy and he said he didn't do it!" It seems my mother had told him, and he confronted Poppy. But Poppy lied. So that was that to them.

This was another kind of silence. You know they know but don't want to know. But I remember my mom saying, "Oh, we can never tell your grandmother—it would kill her." And she would apologize and remind me that I was never going to be alone at Gram's and Poppy's house. So that was their way of dealing with it.

But often Daddy wouldn't be at Gram's and Poppy's. And I would say, "Daddy, you're supposed to be here." And then he would say, "Poppy said he didn't do it." To me it sounded like "You're a liar."

After I told my mother, Poppy stopped touching me. But then he stayed away. He wouldn't talk to me, wouldn't hug me. He was like an icicle. And of course, I felt enormous guilt.

When I was about twelve, something happened with the son of one of my father's friends. Vincent was about eleven years older. I had a huge crush on him. One night we were up watching *Saturday Night Live*—my father and his girlfriend were in another room—and we were sitting on the couch and he started rubbing my legs and inching up toward my vagina. I freaked out and said, "I've got to go to bed."

The next morning, he said, "Please don't tell your dad; I'm sorry." I didn't tell my dad what happened—I told his girlfriend, and she told my dad. My dad put Vincent out. But first there was this trial in the house with Vincent and me, and Vincent started crying. My parents said, "Yeah, what Vincent did was wrong, but you were flirting with him." So, of course, I blamed myself for Vincent crying and being put out, because no one said it *wasn't* my fault.

No one was addressing what Vincent did; no one was talking about what Poppy did.

My grandmother never knew. And that was a huge thing for me, because I was always afraid that I would lose her if she found out.

Gram was very much a free spirit—there was no closing of the bathroom doors, except with Poppy, interestingly enough. She said, "This is your vagina." She was never into nicknames. She was into loving your body, loving nudity, which was in direct opposition from my mother.

My mother thought you should always be covered up. She was very anti-sex. She was into meditation and using sexual energy to attain enlightenment. And my father was into me having sexual pleasure. Not as a preteen, but when I was about fifteen, sixteen. He was into, "You have to make sure that you enjoy sex, because men—that's not going to be their priority." He was saying, "Are you having sex?" And my mother was saying, "You better not be having sex."

My teenage years were not joyous at all. I had started to think and feel like I was attracted to women or girls, but I didn't feel I could talk about it with anybody. It was actually my father who talked to me. And he arranged for me to talk to a Black lesbian. At that point I had a girlfriend, but I wouldn't have said that she was my girlfriend.

In my freshman year at college, I had a breakdown. I felt overwhelmed. Not with college itself, but I think I was just all freaked out. I had just had this relationship with this girl my senior year in high school. I had moved out of my mother's house. It was a lot— and so the dean, at that time a Black woman, sent me to a therapist. And I saw her more consistently than I went to class.

It wasn't until therapy that I began to realize that I didn't flirt with Vincent. My therapist said, "Wait a minute, how old were you?" I told her 12. And she says, "How old was he?" I said, "About twenty-two, twenty-three." She told me, "That's not flirting. You were a child." And then I started dealing with my sexuality.

I have always been on a quest to heal myself in a way that my parents have refused—therapy. They don't think they need it. With my mother it's all about spirituality; my father, it's about politics. But for me, I needed it.

When I was in college, I went on a program to Ecuador. At the time, I was on this mad quest to prove my sexuality. I had thought something was wrong with me. I had a boyfriend at college. We had sex; I enjoyed it, and then we broke up. But after that, I didn't experience any interest in men, women, anything. And so I started freaking out, thinking, "Am I gay?"

In Ecuador, I was with a group of friends and I met this guy selling jewelry. We were talking in Spanish. I was really impressed at how

I was able to converse with him. And he said, "Oh, do you want to go to a hotel and have sex?" And I said yes. I told my friends, and they said, "Oh, go, go!"

So we went to this hotel—this dank place where prostitutes worked. And I paid for the room. When I got in there, I froze; I said, "I don't want to do this." It was clear he wasn't taking no for an answer. But I had broken the rules, because at the school you definitely weren't supposed to be going off with strange men. So I didn't fight or anything—he did use a condom, though when he came out of me the condom wasn't on.

The next morning, when I saw my friends I lied and said, "Oh, it was great." And I spent the whole day at the beach, bathing in the ocean.

Later, I met this other guy and we had consensual sex and I didn't use a condom. I remember being very conscious of that. I didn't care. And I got pregnant. Who knows who the father was?

So I got an abortion. My mother was in a rage.

One friend, who went to the clinic with me, had been working with Women Organized Against Rape. She's the one who told me that I was raped. I didn't even think I was—my thinking was that I said yes, I paid for the hotel room, and I said no, but it wasn't a fight.

In 1990, I came out. I started separating myself from my parents. Everywhere I went, within their circles, I had never had my own identity. I had left school and started doing my own thing.

My mother was disgusted, about the abortion, me dropping out of college, me being a lesbian, all of it. Things didn't get better until she moved abroad for a couple of years, in the mid-1990s, and she started dealing with me as an adult. My dad was very accepting, and he and I became close. Then my grandmother started showing signs of Alzheimer's.

With my grandfather, it was all very complicated. He took care of my grandmother full-time, so she never had to go into a nursing home. My father treated him like a hero. I really resented that.

My speaking out has played a tremendous role for my parents and me. My work—activist work on Black women and rape—has definitely brought us together. Some years ago I got an award for my work, and my dad, stepmother, and my mother, we all went to the ceremony, and I talked about being an incest survivor.

A while after that, my mother called and said: "Every time I hear you say you're an incest survivor, I cringe. And then I remember what you said Poppy did." And when she said that, I just broke down in tears, because I felt like she had enabled me to move out of that "this is a dream" stuff. That was the first time I'd heard anybody acknowledge it.

We began to have these intense conversations—she cried, I cried. And she apologized, for the pain, for the trauma that she caused me.

With my dad, who is very vocal about this issue, I wrote him a letter. I felt like, "You keep wanting to talk about the silence in the Black community; we need to talk about silence in *this* community." But he couldn't deal, and with my grandmother dying, everything came to a head.

I just told him, "I have to talk to you about this." And then he said, "You know, I realized that this happened to you. You wouldn't be talking about this twenty-three years later if it didn't happen." And he said, "I don't know what to do—for the first time in my life I feel completely helpless. I can't handle it." I just needed him to validate it with me.

Just before my grandmother died, something very powerful happened. She had broken her hip, and that was the beginning of the end. I spent the last week of her life with her, and exactly a week before she died—she was not particularly conscious—I told her what had happened. I cried and I told her, "This was the one big thing that I've always wanted to tell you but I've never been able to." And it was so emotional, but it was also freeing. I didn't realize that she was the key. I spent her last days with her in the hospital, massaging her hand and combing her hair and helping her to transition.

It was the closest I had ever come to death, but it was such a healing experience. I really let it go. Or I should say that it was lifted, because when I go to my grandparents' house now, it's full of happy memories. I talk to my grandfather and feel love for him. I'm very clear about what he did and I'm not trying to let him off the hook, but I really feel like, on a metaphysical, spiritual level, she lifted that from me.

It's like my grandmother took it with her when she died.

IRMA (MAYA'S MOTHER)

When Maya told me about the abuse, I didn't believe it. I said, "Oh, maybe you're having a bad dream," because it would always be at night and she would wake up and discover that her grandfather was molesting her. I remember our relationship becoming very difficult. But I thought, "Well, she's becoming an adolescent and she's going through this phase you read about."

There was so much animosity. From the time she was thirteen up until maybe five years ago, and she's now thirty-three. We would have terrible shouting matches and it would never be about this. She would just fly off the handle. Of course I felt like I was a good mother. I did my best. And I would say that to her and that would make her even more angry. Then I would say, "Why are you so angry at me? What didn't I do? What? What? What?" I should have known.

Maya, to her credit, has worked so hard to heal the damage. You know, being in therapy. When she first told me that she was in therapy, as an African American with no history of anybody being in therapy, I didn't understand the level of damage that something like this can do to a young girl.

And because of the incredible healing work that Maya has done against all odds, she can now say she forgives her grandfather. It's just an amazing thing. And thanks in no way to anything that I did to help her. So I'm very ashamed.

The focus of my work is on religion and women. Male religious experts, theologians, have tried to justify oppression of women using religious texts. So in my writings I try to debunk that.

I was always interested in spirituality. I had become very involved with an Islamic group that promoted vegetarianism, meditation, etc. My husband, Allen, wasn't interested, and this added to the breakup of our marriage.

When we broke up, we were both determined to be involved in Maya's life. In some ways having the father wanting to be involved in the child's life can be as difficult as if the father is not involved. So I was struggling with a father whose lifestyle I did not approve of.

In my Islamic group, the whole idea of virginity and chastity is emphasized. Dating was not permitted, and of course, Allen was totally opposed to this. Maya pulled out of the religious community maybe when she was thirteen or fourteen.

So here I've got a vegetarian house, no liquor—from an American point of view, a pretty strict lifestyle. And then Allen goes back to eating meat. I was always saying, "Be sure there's no pork grease in your skillet when you make her eggs," and he would say, "Listen, don't be trying to run my house over here." And it's so ironic that one of the things that I was so concerned about was his male friends and the drinking. And then that would lead to a terrible confrontation. And I'd say, "But she's a girl, Allen, you got to be careful."

I was the first person in my family to go to college and was there on full scholarship. So there was a lot to lose. And I was terrified of losing it because this was my dream come true, little southern girl from the wrong side of the tracks.

Allen and I have a complicated history. I got pulled into the swirling vortex of the Civil Rights Movement when I was a freshman. I met him at a civil rights gathering in Atlanta. We were first colleagues, then became romantically involved and started living together. We later got married. When it became clear that he was going to have to serve jail time, he wanted us to move to Baltimore so he could go to a prison in Maryland, which would be close so his mother could visit.

When his mom became sick with Alzheimer's, she was undergoing treatment and was totally dependent on her husband. I think it's important to remember he's Maya's stepgrandfather, but nonetheless, he carried her home from the hospital. He was involved with her from her birth. I had a lot of respect for him. He seemed like such a nice man, very devoted to Allen's mother. I never saw anything that would make me think he could do something like that.

And I kept saying, "Oh, Maya, it must be a bad dream. Poppy wouldn't do anything like that." Well, after she cried and went on and on, I said, "Something's wrong here." Then I told Allen, "You got to do something."

As I recall, he didn't believe it. So of course I said, "Allen, this is your mama and your family; what can I do? Allen, she can't spend the night over there by herself." And I remember him and me having real difficulty because he said, "Oh, my God, I can't tell my mother, it will kill her." She seemed more of a concern than Maya.

Now as I best remember, after quite a bit of struggle, he said he would speak to Poppy about it. And from what I remember, Poppy denied it. I cannot remember if we made any arrangements for her to go there less. And I don't know whether Allen's speaking to him made him stop.

I don't remember Maya saying more to me about it. But clearly our relationship was terribly impacted, and it was only after she became an adult that it came out that so much of her anger had to do with the fact that I did not protect her.

I thought she was unreasonable. And I thought, "How can you raise a child to hate you and you don't even know why?" I felt, "I love her, but I do not like her." And one of the very difficult periods was after she came out as a lesbian.

When Maya told me, I think I stayed in bed two days. I was in denial. A big part of it was, "This is going to make your life so difficult. You're Black, you're female, that's already difficult. So then you're going to add being an open gay on top of that?" And then she had not finished undergrad. I just thought, "Why is this child destroying her chances for success?"

I'd left college too. I didn't go back till Maya was in high school. But of course, I can say to her, "But look, that was the Civil Rights Movement. Why are *you* not going back?" Now I look back and believe that so much of what was going on was Maya still trying to regain herself from this terrible blow that had seared her soul so deeply.

Knowing what I know now—oh Lord. You'd like to think that you would have done something; I would have been braver. I should have been present with Allen, and at least I could have threatened Poppy personally that I was going to the police if he touched her again, if he even looked at her hard. That I should have done. And I should have let her know that I had done that.

So if I ever have a granddaughter—if she came to me, I would immediately want to, first of all, give her empathy, and get on the case.

It's really sad how we parents can hurt our children when we think we're doing well by them. I had so many blind spots, and did stuff so wrong. And I realize that, and I have to thank Maya for forcing me to deal with it.

Our relationship changed when I began constantly asking her "Why do you hate me? What have I done to you?" And finally she told me.

She told me about the sexual violation, how I didn't believe her, how I took her through the third degree. And oo-wee, she said some stuff to me that was—well, she blew me out of the water. I can't even pull up what was said, but it was painful. We would be on the phone, shouting, screaming. And she could only do it on the phone because I don't believe she could have said these things to me in person.

Her pain was warranted, but I grew up in the Black tradition where children do not say certain things to parents. Many of my friends would say, "This is outrageous! You need to break that relationship off." But I feared for Maya's life, her mental life. And something kept me hanging in there.

When Maya would really go off on me, I would apologize. I would say, "I'm very sorry for what I didn't do, what I did, my ignorance. I can't change anything that happened, but I can tell you that I am very sorry." And often after that there would be maybe five minutes of just silence on the phone and then she might say goodbye. Until the next round. [She laughs.]

We went through this for two or three years. And it just happened gradually. It's been long and arduous and seeing glimmers of light, glimmers of hope.

Today, I think we're friends, most of the time. We have very different lifestyles, different belief systems. But nonetheless, I think there's a real friendship. And I can truthfully say that in addition to loving her, which I always did as a mother, I now like her.

ALLEN (MAYA'S FATHER)

I'm sure that Maya doesn't have anyone she's closer to than me, and vice versa. We're pals, apart from being father and daughter, and we respect each other as intellectual peers.

Our relationship is challenging because we both have such high expectations of each other: how we treat other people, being principled, standing up for what is right. And I was her main supporter— at least in her adult world—when she was struggling with her sexuality.

Maya would always ask, "Dad, how did you know that I was a lesbian?" And I'd say, "I could tell by what you *weren't* doing. Those hormones are raging at sixteen, seventeen. You weren't on the phone with nobody. You weren't talking to anybody. You weren't even trying to sneak around."

It took her mother a while to accept her being a lesbian. For me, it was never an issue.

So Maya and I have this kind of bond, but there was this hole in it. If it's true about being a best friend, then you're supposed to be able to talk to your best friend about something as traumatic as sexual abuse.

From the time I was in high school, I was involved in the Civil Rights Movement. In '65, I went south. Then I began to link the war issues to the civil rights issues, and working with other oppressed peoples.

Irma and I met doing that work, and we went from being friends to husband and wife, to friends again.

Life was complicated when Maya came. Irma had begun a philosophical and metaphysical quest into Islam, and my intellectual pursuits were secular. I mean, she was a Muslim, and basically, I was a Marxist. We broke up in 1974.

Irma was always complaining about my lifestyle and the environment that I had Maya in. I saw it as an attempt by Irma to keep me from being able to see Maya.

If Maya was upset with her mother, then she would kind of hang with me, and then she'd go back and forth. And Maya was very manipulative. She lied. She played her mother and me against each other. Then there were times when both of them, for their own interests, would lie about something. We would have to have a meeting to sort it all out.

The way it was told to me, there was an incident. It was casual. Irma didn't mention it in a way that suggested that anything be done about it. It was kissing, or an attempt to kiss, or something. My antenna went up. I could not tell a behavioral change in either Irma or Maya. Irma didn't stop going over to my parents' house, for example. At my parents', I didn't see any dynamics that would suggest anything.

To this day, there's been nothing I've seen to corroborate that anything happened. Nothing I can use to say, "Ah-hah!"

Except for Irma mentioning it to me, we never talked about this together again. And I didn't talk to Maya about it. I could justify it to myself because Maya was so manipulative in those days. So it was convenient for me to say, "This is just some more BS about me trying to raise my child. Or that's just another wild story."

I have to acknowledge that it took me off the hook from pursuing anything, because let's assume that I did believe it—then what would I have done about it? I would have talked with Maya first and foremost, and then confronted my stepfather.

I know this would have devastated my mother. I have no idea how that would have played out, and I'm not suggesting that that should have been the priority in determining what to do. But I know that had something to do with my response, too.

When my mother got sick, my stepfather and I were taking care of her. There was no pressure on Maya, but she wanted to do what she could. This is how she and I came to talk about the abuse. She told me she felt uncomfortable being over at their house. And it bothered her that we had never resolved my failure to do anything about that issue. That I didn't take any responsibility for her having to carry that alone.

And in fact there were times when something would come up in our conversation about somebody being abused, and either historically, or in a contemporary sense—and Maya would become enraged that I never associated any of that with her. When she became much more conscious of herself, she would refer to being abused. She would refer to being a survivor, and I began to realize that I had buried this thing in my head.

We have built up a faith in each other, a trust. That was the backdrop of our discussion. Now we both know that there's nothing that she and I aren't willing to talk about.

Maya was really angry because she felt that I had been ignoring her reality. Ignoring her pain.

And I told her I was wrong about how I had responded to the abuse. But it was important to go beyond just saying I'm wrong. I talked about ways that I let myself off the hook and still was able to think of myself as a good guy. In retrospect, I said, I don't think I took it serious enough to follow it up.

Now I'm much more aware of the numbers of women who have been abused by a relative or a family friend. Not like some stranger snatching you off the street, but in terms of the most intimate relationships.

I've never talked to my stepfather about it. At the point I had to deal with this, it was so bound up with my mother dying, and Maya and me treated it as something in the past. I must confess, though, that I'm always watching his behavior. I'm always looking for signs.

COMMON RESPONSES TO DISCLOSURE

When an adult discloses childhood abuse, she can no longer bear to carry the secret anymore. She may have given up on the idea of family as anchor and protector and found her own surrogate form of family, sustenance and nurturing. When a child discloses abuse, she is placing her faith in the family trust, distorted though it may be, to keep its children safe. At whatever point she discloses, she is most often met, as Maya was, by a family that mirrors the larger society in questioning her account or even her worth against that of the abuser. In reflecting the attitudes and behaviors we've learned through stereotypes, family members often respond in these ways:

- **Remaining silent.** This can be the most perplexing response to a survivor. After she gathers the courage to tell about the abuse, nothing happens. Acknowledging a disclosure of abuse has consequences that can seem overwhelming. Often what's at play is ignorance—a family member may simply not know what to do and so does nothing. The disclosure could also dredge up long-buried memories of the family member's own abuse, leaving that person incapable of helping another survivor. There could be fear of how people will be affected by the secret (as in Maya's case, of what would happen to her grandmother) or fear of violence or retaliation.

- **Minimizing.** "That's all?" the response might go. "It was only once." Or "At least he didn't . . ." The implication is that the survivor should be grateful that the abuse was not more severe. If we're of the mind that women are for the sexual pleasure of men, that women can be raped with impunity, and that our bodies are not our own, then there is little horror when one of us is violated, and the severity of the violation becomes a factor in determining what a legitimate "victim" is.

- **Blaming.** In Kim's case (Chapter 2), her mother blamed her and put her out of the house for seducing her husband. In a sense, Kim had to sacrifice her relationship with her mother for the abuse to stop. This rejection was so painful that Kim would rather have let the abuse continue than have her life change so drastically.

- **Doubting.** "Are you sure he did that?" "Your father would never do such a thing." These are common ways victims experience others' denial. In Maya's case, her mother made these statements so often that Maya actually began to doubt that her grandfather had done anything.

- **Encouraging to "move on."** Carol, whom we will meet in Chapter 5, saw her family ties disintegrate when her parents pressured her to "get over" her father's abuse. In family counseling, Carol's father acknowledged abusing her. But he minimized the extent, and then asked her why she didn't come around anymore, and why it couldn't be like it was in the old days. Carol, thirty-six, has managed to build a surrogate family of sister-friends in her adopted home of San Francisco. "I've had a desire for my family to be supportive," she says. "I guess mainly because I don't have anyone supporting me in an intimate relationship. But I'm not willing to sacrifice my healing just to be around my family. I don't want to act like what's done is done." And so in her own way and without her family, she has indeed moved on.

Family response and support are not only critical to calming a survivor's fears, quelling anxiety, and stemming emotional and psychological damage, but are also instrumental in getting survivors to recognize that they need help, and then to find the help that is best for them. The next chapter will focus on some of the many roads to recovery.

HELP YOURSELF

Creating the Space to Talk

Some survivors say that one reason they never disclosed a history of sexual abuse is that they were never asked. Even if a parent recognizes unusual behavior, they may find it too difficult to bring up. But often, they simply don't know what to say. Connie, the D.C. sister in Chapter 2 who would unconsciously hold her head down in shame, wishes her mother had found the words to comfort her. "My mother recognized that I wouldn't look up to people," Connie says. "But I don't remember her saying in particular, 'You know, something's wrong. Why is your head always down?' Or 'Why are you so quiet?' I don't remember her opening up room for me to describe what was going on."

Here are ways to start a conversation and to talk about certain behaviors without being intimidating or accusatory. The goal is to focus on the feelings behind the behavior, not changing the behavior itself. Answers may not come the first time the questions are asked, but the process of asking creates a space to answer when the time is right.

- "Why are you so quiet around Uncle Carl?"
- "You never seem to want to visit the Smiths. Why is that?"
- "Is there something wrong between you and your dad?"
- "You're angry right now. Tell me what's upsetting you."
- "I know there's a beautiful body under those baggy clothes. Why do you feel you have to hide it?"
- "Looks like you're troubled by something. Let me help you."
- "Seems like something's weighing you down. When you talk about a problem, you let it go. Let me carry it for you."
- "I know you don't want to talk about it right now, but whenever you're ready, I'll be here to listen."

Responding to the News

Family support is critical to the healing process. If a family member or friend says she was abused, remember that she may have carried this information for years and that her sharing it shows her trust in you. Know that the abuser must be dealt with (see Chapter 7), but first tend to the needs of the survivor. If the abuser still has contact with the survivor, end it immediately. Handle children with special care. See Chapter 5 for specific ways to respond to their disclosures. Try these ways to help an adult who has disclosed she was abused:

- **Listen to what she has to say.** Find a quiet place to talk. She may blurt everything out quickly, or she may be very hesitant. It's important to let her tell at her own pace. Let her know that what she has to say is more important than anything else.

- **Believe her.** Remember that one of the greatest fears of survivors is that they won't be believed or their experience will be minimized. Letting her know that you believe validates her experience.

- **Ask how you can help.** Tell her that you know she's been in pain. Ask her what she needs to deal with it. Ask what she wants to do about the abuser.

- **Encourage her to find outside support.** Suggest calling a local crisis hotline or seeking experienced spiritual guidance or psychological counseling.

- **Reinforce that the sexual abuse was not her fault.** Tell her that you're sorry it happened and that no one had the right to do such a thing. Remind her that no matter what she did, it's the abuser who is at fault.

Don't:

- Judge or criticize
- Blame her or question her actions
- Express doubt about her account
- Defend or make excuses for the person she's accused
- Pressure her to confront the person she's accused
- Suppose what others would have done in her situation
- Compare her experience with someone else's

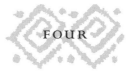

FOUR

"Getting It Out" and Healing

*It's only recently that I've been able to identify myself as a survivor.
It was easier to say I was a drug addict.*

—RAHEMA, who was abused by her brother

IT'S SOMETHING LIKE HAVING A LOW-GRADE FEVER," I REMEMBER MY therapist explaining to me. It was a few months after our initial meeting—after several weekly hour-long sessions in which she gently questioned and probed, and I thought and analyzed and responded. She gave her assessment: My state of depression was just enough to annoy, but wasn't intolerable. "If you weren't looking for it," she said, "you almost wouldn't know it's there." Then she helped me understand what she meant.

For me, depression was so constant that I'd just learned to live with it. It's akin to how, when you're young or foolish or both, you ignore a bad tooth. I admit to having done that—I hate going to the dentist. First you tell yourself that it doesn't hurt *that* badly. Then you say that it doesn't really hurt unless you bite down on it. And then you adapt. You chew all your food on the other side of your mouth. You sip icy soda through a straw positioned so the cold bypasses the tender spot. If it gets worse, you buy something like Orajel and numb the pain. You instinctively learn to live with that tooth. But at some point, the discomfort becomes too much to bear. That's usually when you end up popping Tylenol or Motrin or Bayer until you can get an emergency appointment in the dentist's chair.

That's how many of us deal with the pain of sexual abuse. Some of us end up living with it for so long that we actually get comfortable with it. We may not think of a mental pain as one that needs treating, because we're often able to function in spite of it. We raise our kids, join the PTA, go to work and church, sing in the choir, take care of the house and fall in love, all while knowing it is just beneath the surface. Many physical pains demand immediate attention. But mental distress is not like a broken leg, which forces you off your feet, or fibroids, which cause internal misery. Many of us tend to ignore mental pain; we adapt to it, numb it, or self-medicate. Eventually, though, we have to deal with it. As we know through experience with our physical health, and as I had to learn before I got hip to the dentist, a few things typically happen when you don't work to fix what ails you:

- The pain doesn't go away.
- In fact, it gets worse.
- By the time you end up seeking help, you're in crisis.

I wasn't in crisis when I returned to therapy (I had been disappointed by my first experience, and so I had not gone back for several years), but I was hurting. Like a scar that becomes infected, depression had eased up on me gradually and quietly. I knew there were sore spots, and I either ignored them or tried to cover them up. But every once in a while something would happen that would remind me that the pain was there, just as if I had chomped down on a jawbreaker with a sore tooth. I hated those jarring reminders and realized that to relieve the pain, I needed to find the cause. I knew I couldn't do that on my own, so I asked a trusted friend if she could recommend a therapist. She sent me to a sister psychoanalyst in New York City.

PICTURE OF A WOMAN WITH A PAINFUL PAST

I was wary after my first therapy experience, and I shared with my new therapist that I'd seen a counselor before. We talked about why my discussions with my previous therapist had gone nowhere, and how I wanted this experience to be different. Then we talked about what I wanted out of therapy: to understand why I was so unhappy, especially with myself. We talked about me: how I grew up, whom I trusted, whom I loved, and who loved me. We discussed my relationships with my parents, with my siblings, my husband and son, and with my extended family and friends.

We talked about my work and why it was important to me. We talked about my fierce commitment to justice, where it stemmed from, and how that played out in my volunteer work. We explored what I feared and why, what pleased me and why, what made me angry and why. I opened up and shared, and I laughed and I cried. With her help, I began to see a picture of a woman who had been wounded as a child and carried that hurt into adulthood.

She helped me see that I'd been hurting for so long that I didn't know what it was like *not* to hurt. I had been living with anxiety from having been betrayed by someone I loved, living with anger because my uncle wouldn't admit to what he had done to me, living with unrealistic demands that I'd placed on myself to "make up" for having been sexually abused. My therapist also helped me see that I was suffering from a host of other feelings all too common to abuse survivors: confusion, isolation, guilt, shame (many of these are explored in Chapter 2). I came to realize how I'd buried myself in my work and my commitments as a way to avoid the pain. I explored how I had given up writing, my passion, and had become an editor by profession because it seemed safer to deal with other people's words than to offer mine up for scrutiny. And I learned why I had become a perfectionist and wanted everyone around me to be perfect, too. Anybody who has tried knows that living up to perfection is exhausting and it sets up you and those around you for continuous disappointment and failure.

Most of all, my therapist helped me understand why true happiness and satisfaction seemed out of reach, even though my life included the things that many of us long for: a loving soul mate, a beautiful and healthy child, fulfilling work, and volunteer commitments. No matter how good it all seemed, I found myself living in a constant state of alert, anticipating the worst.

Once we identified some of my issues, we began the difficult work of exploring the causes. Only when I could see clearly the causes and effects could I begin to unlearn unhealthy behaviors that I'd picked up over the years, behaviors that were my ways of avoiding that overwhelming feeling of vulnerability I'd experienced as a girl.

I came to realize that my life does not have to be confined and defined by the parameters of my pain. I learned how to silence that perfectionist's voice in my head that said, "That's not good enough," or "You'll never make it!" whenever I sought to reach for something just beyond my grasp. I decided to step out from the shadows and write again, giving voice to what's in my

Fast Facts

- Thirty-six percent of women with a history of childhood abuse have received a diagnosis of anxiety or depression from a physician within the past five years, compared with 14 percent of women without such a history.[1]
- Among women with a high level of depressive symptoms, more than one of three (37 percent) thought she needed to see a mental health professional in the past year, yet only one of five (20 percent) actually did.
- Forty-six percent of Black American women have a high level of depressive symptoms, compared with 37 percent of White women, 43 percent of Hispanic women, and 41 percent of Asian American women.[2]
- Women who report experiencing difficulty paying for basic needs such as food, telephone service, gas, and electricity are more than twice as likely (68 percent) to experience a high level of depressive symptoms as women who report no such difficulty (32 percent).[3]

soul. And I learned to not be afraid to experience happiness and bask in joy, instead of fretting over things not in my control.

This process wasn't as simple as it seems. Therapy is difficult because the act of dredging up pain is painful in and of itself. Sometimes I'd leave my session exhausted. Sometimes I'd cancel my weekly appointment, feigning a busy work schedule when I simply wanted to avoid unhappy memories. But ultimately I made a commitment to continue, because I wanted to heal.

PATHS TO HEALING

No two paths to healing are the same. Your experiences and needs are far different from mine. You may be in a low-grade state of depression like I was, or you may be like Lori, the Detroit hairstylist we met in Chapter 2, who was in crisis, or you may be somewhere in between. You may find that sifting through your past to solve problems today is too tedious; you simply may want to zero in on changing negative thoughts and behaviors. You might prefer the camaraderie of a group to the one-on-one of individual therapy, or a holistic approach to a traditional one. You might embrace artistic forms of healing, like dance, art, or journaling, instead of or in addition to talk therapy. You might find it easier to turn to a spiritual healer you know or to a new mental health professional from whom you have nothing to hide.

We have historically turned to our own support systems—girlfriends, sister circles, family, and clergy among them—but for many of us the problems associated with being sexually abused run far too deep for untrained experts to help us tackle them in a meaningful way.

I am not advocating psychotherapy for everyone; the path you choose is a decision you must make based on your own needs and resources. But I encourage you to seek relief. The majority of survivors I interviewed found that traditional talk therapy helped them regain control of their lives, but some have recovered through other means, like the arts and self-help. The actual method is not as important as finding a healthy way to lessen the depression, anxiety, stress, and other problems stemming from sexual abuse. If you have thoughts of suicide or want to harm yourself or those around you, seek professional help immediately. There are several hotline and help line contacts in the Resources section of this book.

Like many African Americans, you may think that therapy is not for you because you're not "crazy" or "weak." If so, consider that we all have our issues and that we can choose to do something about them or choose not to. It may feel comfortable remaining where you are, if only because you are familiar with the place you are in. For some of us, changing the tune is more frightening than singing the same old miserable song. But imagine taking on the challenge of change and composing a new score for your life. Imagine feeling entitled to joy and then going after it, grabbing hold of it. Imagine how it would feel *not* to be depressed, angry, bitter, anxious, or overly critical of yourself and those you love. Healing is a sense of wholeness that engulfs and overshadows even the pain of your past. With help, it is within your reach. Consider these common options:

Fast Facts

- Single women with children—widowed, divorced, separated, and those who never married—are more likely to suffer from a high level of depressive symptoms than are married women with children (51 percent versus 38 percent).[4]
- Women who lack a source of social support when feeling stressed, overwhelmed, or depressed are nearly twice as likely as those who have support to report high levels of depressive symptoms (68 percent versus 36 percent).[5]

TALK THERAPY

Individual Therapy

Talk therapy, or psychotherapy, has been a mainstay of mental health care for the last century. It is most often used to treat problems like anxiety and depression, and to help people reach specific goals. The main benefits of talk therapy, says Maelinda Turner, the San Francisco social worker, is to begin the process of healing. "It's for people not to feel isolated, to feel supported and validated," she says, "particularly in sexual abuse cases, where the family doesn't believe you." Turner, a disability care manager for a managed-care company, is researching depression in the workplace. At any given time, one employee in twenty is experiencing depression, which, if left untreated, disrupts family and personal life.[6] Talk therapy includes the Freudian analytical approach, which involves exploring the past, the conscious and the unconscious, and the increasingly popular cognitive approach, which is shorter-term and more like coaching to reach specific goals.[7] Many therapists practice a combination of the two, along with other techniques that include behavioral therapy, which zeroes in on changing behaviors that lead to depression. In talk therapy, a person meets with a trained professional to discuss issues, concerns, and goals. That service provider can be a psychologist, psychiatrist, social worker, or other degreed and licensed counselor. Many of us turn to members of the clergy for counseling, and if this is what you want to do, make sure the person you choose is trained to deal with issues related to sexual abuse. If the clergy member knows other family members involved, consider whether he or she may be biased. For a host of reasons that we explored in Chapter 1, including embarrassment and a deep mistrust of a majority White medical profession, Blacks have been slow to embrace traditional therapy. When we do, we often find ourselves sitting across from a counselor who hasn't a clue about the complexities of our culture, our history, and our challenges, and who can only see our problems solely from a White or middle-class perspective. Since the late '60s experts have developed multicultural approaches to therapy that incorporate the values, customs, and traditions of non-Whites. One of these, the African-centered approach, builds upon basic tenets we have inherited from our African ancestors, including our embrace of spiritual thinking and living, our emphasis on the collective "we" versus the individual "I," and our commitment to supporting our communities. Time and time again, Turner finds these tenets among her Black clients. "There's that African American belief that you're never given anything you can't handle," she says. "Well, with help, you can handle it. But when we come through on the other side, we tend to look at the kind of spiritual leader that makes us, and how we can help other people. With us, we're trying to see the bigger picture—not just why did this happen, but what am I supposed to learn from this." One excellent resource for understanding African-centered healing is the book *The Psychology of Blacks,* by Thomas A. Parham, Joseph L. White, and Adisa Ajamu (see Bibliography). By incorporating our culture and our values into their work, counselors of any race can provide mental health care in a way that is more relevant to our lives.

Group Therapy

Group therapy provides the opportunity to connect with other survivors under the guidance of a facilitator who is a trained counselor. "Group" is not just about commiserating or piling on one another's misery. Nor is it a contest to see whose experience was worse. It is about finding comfort in the company of those who have shared a similar history and who are working to overcome similar issues. Groups can range from a few people to more than a dozen. Each session may be two hours or more, to allow enough time for members to talk. Group leaders raise questions and encourage open, uninhibited give-and-take among members. Groups allow members to question and challenge one another, with the guidance of the facilitator. Groups may be organized by sex, by experience, by age, or by all or none of the above. At the Institute for Family Services in Somerset, New Jersey, the founder, Rhea Almeida, leads groups that include men and women from a range of racial and ethnic backgrounds. A sexual abuse survivor might find herself sitting next to a domestic violence survivor and responding to a recovering domestic or sexual offender who discusses his or her issues. This unorthodox mix is Almeida's way of helping people seek common bonds in ways other than their victimization. "Typically in mental health, if you're an incest victim, they'd put you in an incest victims' group," she says. "If you're a battered woman, they'd put you in a battered women's group. I've found that that kind of separation only further isolates clients."

Watching a session one night through a one-way mirror, I saw the discomfort of recovering offenders who listened with the rest of the group as a young woman shared a detailed and painful letter to her father describing the effects of the years of his sexual and emotional abuse. (Clients are aware they may be watched; they sign consent forms acknowledging as much.) I also heard members challenge one of the newest members, who was still blaming his wife's "attitude" for the beatings he gave her. "We know that isolation is a major factor in how perpetrators operate as well," Almeida says. Some groups require that members be in individual therapy in addition to group. This ensures that each member has one-on-one help dealing with her or his particular issues.

Family Therapy

Sometimes it helps to work out issues when all the affected parties are in the same room. Janet Davis, a social worker at the Northside Center for Children, a Harlem community mental health center that also treats adults, says when she thinks an adult client is ready, she will ask if she or he wants to invite family members to attend a session. Davis may start with the client and Mom, or she may ask that up to five people join the client. These gatherings are rarely easy, but Davis helps family members begin to explore current relationships and interactions as well as past behaviors and experiences that are too difficult to talk about on their own. "First you get people saying, 'This happened years ago. Why do you want to bring it up now?'" Davis says. Before the meeting she will often call family members or invite them to call her. In cases involving sexual abuse, she tries to explain that the "this" that happened years ago is affecting their daughter's or sister's ability to function today. Often, she says, the family is already aware that the client is having difficulty, and many know why. So reluctantly, and with her encouragement, they come. "The biggest hurdle is trust," Davis says. "Nobody wants outsiders to know their business, and nobody wants to be judged." In a family session, Davis helps survivors verbalize their experience of abuse and how they've been affected, and then she encourages family members to respond. She'll ask parents, for instance, "Are you surprised that your child is saying that?" Often, Davis says, parents are more embarrassed than surprised. She has toned down shouting matches and asked disruptive people to leave. She has let silent family members remain silent, because she knows they can hear what's being said. Eventually, she pulls them in. Family therapy may last a few sessions or more, depending on the rate of progress. Usually she sees the client once a week and the client with the family every other week. Throughout it all, Davis makes sure to support the survivor. "People often charge that it's all the survivor's fault, that everything was fine before this was dug up, but in reality everybody knows it wasn't fine. People tend to think they have the perfect family, but I haven't come across the perfect family yet."

Couples Therapy

Many survivors of child sexual abuse need to learn how to have intimate relationships based on trust and mutual respect, as opposed to the fear, powerlessness, and domination that they once experienced. Because child sexual abuse often involves emotional and sexual intimacy found in traditional adult couple relationships, as one expert writes, survivors may find it difficult to form close relationships in adulthood.[8] Partners of survivors often need support, as they have to deal with the effects of the abuse, too. A survivor may struggle to communicate her needs, and her partner may not know how to help. She may lash out in anger one day, then sulk in sadness the next, and he may feel confused and overwhelmed by her unpredictable behavior and needs. Or if she has not shared her history of abuse, her partner may think he is to blame for her emotional distance or lack of interest in sex. He may not be aware that something he does or says, or even the way he smells or touches her, could remind her of an abuser or an act of violation. Without open, honest communication, a relationship can collapse under the weight of the stress associated with abuse. Many healers say that relationship problems are one of the most frequently reported complaints of survivors seeking counseling. Unlike individual therapy, which focuses on self-understanding and personal growth, couples therapy focuses on helping partners resolve issues that block emotional and physical intimacy between them. For Karen, thirty-eight, a Wichita, Kansas, sister who found healing through bibliotherapy, and her husband, Erroll, forty, talking about making love was the only way they could do so. They met a few years ago, and the attraction was instant. They married less than six months later. As their initial excitement settled into routine and familiarity, Karen began to withdraw. When Erroll pressed for an explanation, Karen shared some of her memories of being abused by her stepfather from ages twelve to sixteen. Though they had no professional counseling, through communication each came to understand the other's needs and expectations. This is what worked for them.

> **Karen:** When we first started dating, we were talking about what happened the first time we did it. And I told Erroll, well, I didn't have the luxury of choosing who I was going to be with. He was angry, but because his mother is a survivor, and he is a product of that, I think it made him more sensitive to what I was going through, and how his mother probably felt. And so that just opened up a whole other round of conversation for us. It started with me performing oral sex on my stepfather. He was an alcoholic, and he

would come home drunk from work and wake me up in the middle of the night saying, "Come on." And we would go into the kitchen area. Everyone else would be asleep. Imagine walking into a room and seeing it prepared. Blankets on the floor. I remember that many times, he'd have me in my mother's—in their bed. He would be very forceful with me. It wasn't, "If you do this then I'll get you this new bike," because we had all of that already. It was really more of, "If you say something, then I'll hit your mother," or, "I'll hurt you and your brother or sister," or "I'll have somebody pour acid in your face." Somehow I disconnected with it. At some point, I decided, "He can have my body, but not my mind." I had to talk to Erroll about this. That first year was really rough for us, but that's why God gives you that extra challenge, to force your hand. Because if I didn't have him in my life, I would probably continue not to allow a person into my space. I'd still want to be in control. In my marriage, I have to allow myself to be vulnerable. Allow myself to let somebody get into that spot that makes me uncomfortable. My husband loves to see me walk around naked, but I'm still a little insecure with that. I went through a period where I didn't want anyone to look at me. You have to find a way to share that intimacy. You should be enjoying your husband because he's your husband, and you have to fight back memories and thoughts of what happened to you. You have to say, "Well, this is not the person that did this to me." I'm having to remind myself that it's okay for me to look like this. And it's okay for him to be attracted to me. But sometimes I just have to say, "Today is my day." And he knows that means don't come trying to rub on me. Don't come trying to talk me into anything, because that means I need my space. And it's really empowering, too, to be able to say, "Well, no, I don't want to." Or, "Tonight is not the night." And to have him just say, "Okay."

Erroll: When Karen told me, I viewed it as something that had happened and it was over. But I had no idea that there were still scars. At first I felt rage. I thought, "Why don't I go and find this person and do something physically to him?" And then I thought, "Well why don't I just go and humiliate him and tell his job they have a child molester in their employment?" It's a natural reaction. But I had to realize, I'm not helping our situation. In fact, I'm putting more strain on the relationship, because she's thinking, "Oh, if I hadn't told him, he wouldn't be feeling like this." When we first got together, I thought, "Oh, the sex is pleasing. Room for growth, but I'm willing to commit for the rest of my life for this." But when I started to experience what I took as rejection, I could not understand it. But I soon realized that one of the reasons that she had been single for so long was because she was not willing to share about her past. The reason we've been able to be together this long is because we committed so early. And once we started talking, she mentioned, "When I was younger I used to be awakened in the middle of the night." I now know I can never wake her up in the middle of the night, regardless of what I'm feeling. And when I tell my wife, "You're beautiful," I need to remember that, yes, she may be beautiful, but he used to say to her, "You think you're beautiful now. Let's see when I pour some battery acid on your face." Although you may tell your mate, "I love you," "I love you" may have a negative association with it, because in some cases the perpetrator may have told her that. One time I suggested we watch an adult video. She ended up writing me a letter about how she couldn't watch those things because they remind her of her past. One of the things that survivors should know is that when you have a significant other, if you want that relationship to move forward, then share with them what you've gone through. The specifics can be given on a need-to-know basis. By letting a person know what you're going through, they're more likely to put their agenda aside and help. But if we don't know what you're going through, all we see is rejection. And rejection is powerful; it's devastating. One of the things that Karen said to me was that as she was being assaulted, she had to remove herself, subconsciously, from it, so that she didn't express or reflect anything that would encourage it. And so the fact that she's able to share anything intimately is a tremendous accomplishment, so I'm not pushing the issue.

FINDING THE RIGHT THERAPIST

You can find mental health counselors and therapists through a variety of resources. But first, consider your priorities. Do you prefer individual or group, or both? Must the provider be African American? Male or female? Should the provider be in your health insurance network? (Many private therapists do not accept insurance.) Can the therapist be in a community clinic? How much time can you commit? What can you afford?

As I did, you might start by asking a trusted friend if she or he knows of a counselor. Or if you're uncomfortable with that approach, look in your phone book or on the Internet for a local rape or sexual assault crisis center. Also look under "community services," "mental health," or "health and human services" in your government listing for city- or county-run services. Several national organizations, like the YWCA, act as a clearinghouse for local providers. The Rape, Abuse & Incest National Network (RAINN) offers twenty-four-hour crisis intervention and can refer you to a nearby rape crisis center. You can also try VOICES (Victims of Incest Can Emerge Survivors) and the Association of Black Psychologists for referrals (all contact information is in the Resources section of this book).

Some counselors are covered by health insurance; you should check with your insurer to determine what kind of referral you may need. Many private counselors who are not part of insurance plans offer sliding scales or flexible-payment options depending on your income. Many community clinics provide mental health care covered by Medicaid and Medicare. Some programs are free of charge.

Understand that the therapist you choose will only be able to guide you; she or he will not give you answers. "You must bring to the table a willingness to understand why you're there and what you want to get out of the process," Turner says. "The therapist may give you insight and tasks to do, but you're the judge on how you're able to heal." To see if you're a good match with a therapist, you should interview your counselor. Turner remembers one client who brought a list of questions for her first visit. If you're uncomfortable, take a trusted friend to your first meeting. Ask questions like these:[9]

- How long have you been counseling?
- What is your educational background and training?
- Are you currently licensed to practice therapy?
- Do you have a certification or special expertise in working with survivors of childhood sexual abuse?
- How many sexual abuse clients have you worked with?

- What kind of therapy do you practice (for example, cognitive, analytical, behavioral)?
- Do you think sex with a client can be therapeutic? (If the answer is yes, leave immediately.)
- Is there a contact number where I can reach you during off hours in case of emergency? (If the person is inaccessible, find another therapist.)
- Will you give me books to read or exercises to do?
- What is your fee?
- How open are you to alternative forms of healing? (Many people combine traditional therapy with other methods, including art therapy and bodywork. If you want to pursue these other therapies, make sure your talk therapist is receptive to them.)
- How open are you to spirituality and the metaphysical? (As Turner says, "Among African Americans, there's more of a dependence on prayer and a recognition that there is a higher force. If I'm having dreams and my ancestors are talking to me, I want to be able to bring it up without being minimized or discriminated against.")
- How will I know our work is done?
- What is your termination process?

After the meeting, Turner says, here are some questions to ask yourself:

- Was I comfortable? Can I be honest with this person? (Therapy is based on trust, and feeling you can share your most intimate concerns, hopes, and fears is the foundation of the work that you will do.)
- Did the therapist seem interested in what I had to say?
- Was the therapist open to my questions? (Avoid anyone who seems put off by your interview.)
- Did the therapist seem to respect my racial and ethnic background, my gender and sexual identity, my educational background and economic standing? Does how much I can pay for services matter?
- Could I challenge this person if I feel my needs aren't being met? (You must not feel intimidated. One sister I interviewed was not satisfied with her counselor but did not want to end her visits for fear of making the counselor angry. Turner described that dynamic as "an imbalance of power.")

A no to any of these questions means to move on. Similarly, here are some warning signs that your counselor is not acting in your best interest. If your counselor does the following, leave immediately:

- Tells you what to do or how you should feel
- Questions or challenges your truthfulness
- Suggests that sex with a client can be therapeutic, or that child/adult sex can be beneficial
- Belittles you or puts you in a situation in which you feel violated or victimized, either sexually or emotionally
- Falls asleep or shows a general lack of interest

If your worst fear is that your therapy will go on forever, you'll be glad to know that counseling does come to an end. Most managed-care programs cover between three and twelve sessions, typically with a "termination period" evaluating and culminating your progress. But when the root of the problem is sexual abuse, Turner says, she recommends longer-term treatment. "Because the trauma is so intense, you generally need at least a year." You and your therapist can determine the length of time that is right for you. And how do you know you're ready to end? "When you feel you have the skills and tools to walk on your own," Turner says. "Therapy is all a journey of healing. And each person you know is a part of that journey. Sometimes you're on the train with the therapist, sometimes you're on with a friend. Sometimes a new person you meet helps take you further. Therapy can only take you so far, and at some point you should be able to say, 'I now have what I need to walk on my own.'" While you may not feel progress overnight with most therapies, you will come to a point where you can look back and see how far you've come.

OTHER THERAPIES

For some of us, talking about our problems is not enough. Or it's simply not the best way we express ourselves. For the artist, the writer, the musically inclined, or the person interested in the metaphysical, other therapies can be an alternative or a complement to traditional talk. The ultimate goal is to acknowledge that trauma happened and has affected you, and then to release it and move on. Turner says that alternative therapies are particularly helpful when dealing with incidents that happened when you were young and couldn't even articulate or understand what was happening. You can find alternative therapists in hospitals, community health centers, disability-care facilities, drug rehab centers, correctional facilities, nursing homes, and schools as well as in private practice. Many alternative therapists work in teams with medical professionals and traditional psychotherapists. Before you begin working with them, ask about their licensing and accreditation. Here are some other popular therapies:

Creative Therapies

It has been widely documented that creative expression can be therapeutic. Using creativity helps access emotions in ways that you may not be able to reach intellectually. "It's easy to be just inside your head," says Turner. "When dancing, writing, creating music, you reach a whole different level of the intuitive process." Turner has found arts therapy to be very effective in working with young survivors or those who don't have the vocabulary to adequately express themselves. For Tracey, a thirty-year-old Chicagoan who was repeatedly molested by her father for about ten years, dance proved to be not just an avocation but a lifeline. After graduating from college, she switched her focus from history to dance and, through a master's program, pursued her own form of therapy. "I really was interested in the art of dance and how it heals," she says. Early on it was a struggle. "I don't get this comment so much from my teachers now, but they would constantly tell me, 'Stop thinking. Stop thinking!' They would see me trying to figure out the moves. I had to learn that the process of dancing is really surrendering to the body, and as a survivor, it was so hard for me to surrender. Because I just didn't feel safe in my body. I felt like my body betrayed me because although I was under attack, my body responded as if I was enjoying it. I had done traditional therapy, and found that incredibly helpful. Therapy helps you put words to your feelings, but as we are all mind, body, and spirit, it doesn't make sense to leave any one part out. Dance unifies the body, the mind, the voice, the emotions. This is also important in the sense of telling your story—externalizing it and putting it out there." When we last spoke, Tracey was choreographing a dance about healing for a community arts program. She was also working on her doctorate in dance.

Dance Officially, dance therapy is the use of movement to help improve emotional, mental, social, and physical wellness. Professional dance therapists help clients "integrate knowledge of body, movement and expressive spirit with healing skills of counseling, psychotherapy and rehabilitation."[10]

Art   Through the use of art media and the creation of images, this therapy helps people become more aware of themselves and others, to cope with symptoms, stress, and traumatic experiences, according to the American Art Therapy Association. The profession emerged in the 1930s with psychiatrists taking an interest in the artwork done by patients and educators, noting the emotional and symbolic messages of children's spontaneous artwork. Therapists are professionals trained in art and therapy, with knowledge of "human development, psychology, clinical practice, spiritual, multicultural and artistic traditions."[11]

Music   Musical ability isn't necessary to benefit from music therapy, in which music making and passive listening are used to help improve physical, mental, or social functioning. Music's healing influence dates at least to the writings of Aristotle and Plato, according to the American Music Therapy Association, but the twentieth-century discipline of music therapy began after World War I, when community musicians both amateur and professional went to veterans' hospitals around the country and played for vets suffering physical and emotional trauma. Today's music therapy is focused on the individual, as music is selected and sessions are designed based on each client's preferences, circumstances, needs, and treatment plan.[12]

Writing and Journaling   A common form of therapy, keeping a regular diary of interactions, reflections, and emotions, is often an integral part of a therapeutic process. Indeed, in *The Courage to Heal,* one of the most popular books for sexual abuse survivors, writing exercises occur throughout the book. In a typical psychotherapy treatment plan, Turner may give a client a writing exercise. "I may have you write about your experience, but after a few pages, I'll ask you to stop writing about it and write about what feelings come up for you as you write about a particular issue. And then we talk about it."

Eye Movement Desensitization and Reprocessing (EMDR)

A treatment that has emerged since the late 1980s, EMDR has been used to help survivors of trauma, including victims of sexual and domestic violence, crime victims, veterans, and those suffering from addictions, phobias, depression, and self-esteem issues. In EMDR, a practitioner has the client remember and discuss a traumatic event, including the negative physical and emotional sensations they experienced at the time. While recalling the event, the client visually follows the quick back-and-forth rhythms of the therapist's hand or object. Some therapists incorporate flashing lights or repetitive sounds as well. The process "focuses not just on a person's troubling feelings, but on the thoughts, physical sensations, and behaviors related to those feelings as well," explains Francine Shapiro, the psychologist who conceived and developed EMDR.[13] The eye movements are thought to desensitize the client to the negative emotions and sensations. The next step is to "reprocess," or replace negative thoughts like "I felt powerless" at the time of the event with positive ones like "I am now in control."

Hypnotherapy

Clinical hypnosis is used to bring a client to an altered level of awareness or consciousness, to treat physical or psychological ailments. In a hypnotic trance, the client's subconscious is open and responsive to suggestions that can reduce physical pain, change behavior, improve memory and concentration, and lessen phobias and anxiety.[14] In psychotherapy, hypnosis can help a client become relaxed and comfortable enough to tackle difficult memories and experiences. Hypnosis, whose roots have been traced to ancient civilizations, is accepted by national psychological, medical, dental, and other professional organizations. Hypnotherapists stress that treatment does not cause clients to turn over control of their consciousness or mind. Many practitioners may identify themselves as "certified," but to find someone qualified to treat your condition, the American Society of Clinical Hypnosis advises that you contact only licensed mental or physical health care professionals who will use the therapy in accordance with their own licensing and training laws. The society provides a referral service through its Web site: www.asch.net/referrals.asp.

Massage or Bodywork

Massage and bodywork, hands-on manipulation of the muscles and soft tissues of the body, was once considered pampering for the elite, done in fancy spas. But massage is becoming more and more popular among the masses as a therapeutic response to stress and anxiety, injury and pain. Once on a trip home from Brazil, I saw a steady stream of weary travelers lining up for ten-minute seated massages right in the airport waiting area. In addition to relieving stress, massage is a part of many physical rehabilitation programs and eases conditions like lower back pain and arthritis. There are hundreds of types of therapeutic massage, including Swedish (one of the most popular), sports, and prenatal. Many methods used today have both Eastern and Western origins. Shiatsu, acupressure, and reflexology come from the Eastern sources. It is often through massage that clients can begin to address issues related to abuse, says Chimene Green, a sister in Columbia, South Carolina, who is a bodywork specialist. Perhaps it is the simple act of touch ("The body remembers every injury," she says) that connects them with their past. "People will come because they're under stress, or their body aches," Green says. But as a session is under way, she will see other issues emerge. "I might feel a sense of sadness, or pain." She doesn't ask questions or probe, but through her work tries to create a space in which a client might open up. And sometimes they do. "People have so many layers of armor that it takes time. Then you come almost to the soft part and the tears will flow. Sometimes they won't even say anything but you'll see a difference and you recognize that something just happened on the table." Other times, she says, "We'll just start talking and they'll say, 'Do you have a moment?' And that moment turns into more talking than massage—just a connection of the souls."

Reiki The term *reiki* is typically translated as "universal life-force energy." Said to be an ancient, spiritual form of healing from Japan (though it is not connected to any religious belief), Reiki is best described as a transmission of healing energy through the hands. The practice, which is done worldwide according to the International Association of Reiki Professionals, can ease tension and stress and promote spiritual, physical, emotional, and mental well-being.[15] In a typical hour-long session, a Reiki practitioner places his or her hands on a client's body, following a specific sequence of positions. No massage is involved. The movement helps direct energy where it is most needed. Clients remain fully clothed and can recline or sit upright.

Bibliotherapy Bibliotherapy, the use of books to help people solve problems, is an old, familiar concept and, says one source, can be traced to the days of the first libraries in Greece.[16] Studies show that bibliotherapy is most effective as a complement to other therapies. Reading self-help, nonfiction, and even fiction works can be self-selected or guided by a counselor. For Karen, the Wichita sister, bibliotherapy was a source of information about dealing with sexual abuse. But then it became one of inspiration. "I've not done any therapy—well, not like sitting on somebody's couch," says Karen, who was abused by her stepfather for four years. "But I've worked out things by reading and thinking about how they relate to me. Even when I was younger, I'd read what books I could find. I would write poems or write my thoughts and feelings. And then I did a book report on sexual abuse. The information I read was all so negative about the way these girls turn out— that they become prostitutes, or they use drugs, or they use alcohol to deal with the situation. I decided that wasn't the route that I wanted to take. I wanted to be positive, to make something out of myself. For everything that they said negative, I decided to do the opposite."

STAGES OF PROGRESS

The preceding sections describe some of the more popular therapeutic options; this list could go on and on. Before you consider moving forward, think about which best suits your needs, and how you receive ideas and express yourself. Know that whatever your path toward healing, on your way you will pass through stages that are similar to those of other survivors. Looking back at my progress, I know I went through three stages that I call acknowledgment, understanding, and action. Through the stories of three women, we will explore some of the many ways that survivors pass through these stages, and the kinds of issues that they face along the way.

Acknowledgment

Before you can begin to heal, you must first acknowledge the source of your pain. This step is the first toward recovery. For some, even before they can acknowledge, they must *remember* that they were abused. About eight years ago, with the help of a therapist, Rahema, thirty-four, a Baltimore sister who works in city government, began to envision scenes of her own abuse. She was about three when it started, and she remembers events vaguely. "What I do know is that I had a special relationship with one of my older brothers and that I was his favorite and I was special only to him," she says. One therapist speaks of "body memory," the ability to recall how certain areas of the body were affected, but not actual incidents of abuse. If you have body memory, claim it as real. Acknowledgment of abuse often comes after a struggle to move beyond denial and perhaps others' urgings to "get over it." Acknowledgment is also telling another person about it. Having someone bear witness to the source of your pain can be remarkably liberating.

Understanding

Once you acknowledge the abuse, you need to understand what happened and how it affects your life today. Whatever form of therapy you embrace, this new information gives you a foundation from which to do your work. To help understand your experience, ask yourself: "How often did the abuse happen? What was involved? Who was the abuser and how close was I to him or her? In what ways did it affect my life, and how do I want to change that?" Lori, the Detroit hairstylist we met in Chapter 2, recalls how her father's beatings during his attacks when she was a child led her to becoming overextended as an adult. "When I would say no, bad things would happen to me," she says. This stage of recovery, which includes many phases itself, can be extremely difficult and should be entered with the help of a qualified mental health professional. As you undergo counseling, consider the ways in which you responded to abuse, and how your life has been shaped by those responses. Then prepare to move through the next phase: untangling the effects of abuse from your life.

Action

Knowing how abuse affected my life, I sought ways to undo the damage. I devoured information on abuse survivors. I wrote about it, sharing my experience and offering ways that other survivors could break their silence and get help. I then decided to write this book. Many people who have experienced sexual or physical violence feel compelled to do something to counteract the effects of abuse. Some people confront those who victimized them, detailing the pain they caused. Some decide to forgive the abuser, or at least release their hatred for that person (I will address confronting and forgiving in Chapter 8). Some, vowing to protect other children in their family, identify abusers to other relatives. Some become activists, joining organizations and lending their voices to antiviolence causes. Some go into healing or protecting professions, becoming physicians, nurses, police officers, social workers. One such person is Shantel, a thirty-eight-year-old social worker whose mother's boyfriend violated her for years. Now Shantel counsels children in her city's social services department. When an abused person takes action, she moves not only from victim to survivor, but also from survivor to *healer*. Many healers who are survivors acknowledge that playing an active role in stopping violence is a way through which they themselves continue to heal. As Shantel says, "I've learned much about myself from working with victims." Her next move: counseling juveniles who have committed sexual offenses. As you read about these women's experiences, consider the ways that they moved through the stages of acknowledgment, understanding, and action, and where you are as well.

RAHEMA'S STORY: FACING THE MEMORIES

Rahema is a rising administrator in one of Baltimore's social services agencies. In her power suits, her pumps, and her striking African-inspired jewelry, this thirty-seven-year-old mother of four is the epitome of the professional woman. You would never know that sixteen years ago, she was a closet junkie, as she describes it, making the grades at school while piling up arrest warrants for shoplifting or stealing, and dancing with death by sleeping with men to feed her habit.

She grew up in a household full of addicts. In her family of seven older siblings and their single mother, four were on drugs, three were alcoholics. Chaos reigned, and when there wasn't self medication, there was mayhem and misery. One brother was murdered outside their housing project just before Rahema was born, two brothers died of AIDS, and a sister succumbed to cancer before her fortieth birthday. Rahema's first taste of alcohol came at eleven. Cocaine? That came at fifteen, courtesy of a sister who was dating drug dealers. "I was a dope fiend at seventeen years old," she says.

For years Rahema lived with deep, gnawing feelings of fear: "Fear of intimacy, fear of not being good enough, fear of overachieving, fear of underachieving, fear for my safety and, most of all, fear of not being loved." Fear, she says, "became a living, breathing being inside of me that dictated my actions and determined my behavior. I have made at least twenty years' worth of bad decisions because of this one emotion."

Just as shoplifting was her escape from poverty, alcohol and drugs were her escape from fear. But every so often that fear would swoop in on her, clouding her vision and her judgment, and leading her to run. In 1988, after several failed tries, she finally decided to confront her addictions. In doing so she explored the roots of those fears: long-buried memories of sexual abuse by one of her brothers. Allowing herself to remember led Rahema to reclaim "that terrified little girl" who was left behind at age six.

"To date I still don't have a vocabulary or clear memory of the acts committed against me," she says, "but I have all the feelings and behaviors of a survivor." She does remember the special relationship she had with one of her brothers, and that "I was his favorite." She began to explore these memories in therapy, after detox. And then she began to get her life back.

It was a life that was almost lost. At her lowest point, Rahema found herself married, a new mother struggling to stay clean, a college student with a part-time job, watching her husband being carted off to prison on drug-related charges. With no support or script for living an addiction-free life, she says, "I just kind of gave up. I wound up back on drugs real heavy this time. I gave my daughter to my mother, quit my job, dropped out of school, and took to the streets. I was twenty-one and just out there, stealing, getting high, robbing jewelry stores, getting in a world of trouble. I am so grateful I'm not dead."

And there was sex. "Sleeping with drug dealer guys that I would have never, ever otherwise thought about. One guy started beating me really bad. Sent me to the hospital with a busted lip. I was confusing sex terribly, sex for money, sex for love, sex for attention. I was the kind of girl who would let you feel me up in the hallway at twelve or thirteen. I remember a guy feeling me up and ejaculating all over my leg in the stairwell in the housing projects. I had no value, no concept that this is not something that girls do."

She was high on heroin when she learned that one of the men she'd slept with had died of AIDS. That scared her enough to get tested. But to be tested, she was told, she had to be clean. She had tried before, but this was the first time that she'd done so in about five years. She was twenty-five and remembers it well. "It was Easter Sunday and I left my daughter with my mom, in her dress and her shoes, and I said, 'I'm going away, baby, to get myself together.' I stayed there for weeks, detoxing from heroin and cocaine. That is where I first heard what we call the message of recovery."

April 24, 1989, is the day Rahema celebrates as her release from drugs. When she left detox she moved in with a sister who was an alcoholic. Friends from Narcotics Anonymous told her that was no place to be and helped her find an apartment and a job with a city outreach agency for recovering addicts. She got pregnant by a recovering addict and had a son. Her children stayed with her mother as Rahema tried to build a life. A few years into recovery, her sponsor saw her wavering and suggested therapy. "She said,"

Rahema remembers, "'I can bring you the message of recovery outside or I can bring it to you in jail. Which will it be?'" Rahema chose therapy.

She also chose therapy because she knew it was time to face her fears. "I was having all these recurring feelings and I was afraid to mention them because I thought I would be called crazy. Two of my sisters had mental illnesses; one was bipolar. My brother—the one who abused me—used to do cocaine and run through the neighborhood naked and people would tease me at school. I always felt, 'I don't want to be like those crazy people.'"

She found a therapist through a community mental health program that provided services on a sliding fee scale. The therapist was a White Jewish woman. Across the chasms of race, religion, and class, they managed to connect. "I would say something like 'You don't understand what it's like to grow up like I did,'" Rahema says, "and she would say, 'I know what it's like to be angry, to be disappointed.'"

In her second session, the abuse came up. "I remember she was going through my family and I was talking about each sister and brother. And I got to this brother and said, 'Well, we were special.' She said, 'Why?' I couldn't answer. But things started to click. We've estimated that it was between the ages of two or three up to about eleven. I remember him giving me gifts all the time, jewelry, things like that. I have vague memories of being in bed with him or him putting me on top of him. Of the coarseness of his hair rubbing against me. For a long time I couldn't give a man a blow job. I didn't have orgasms. Sex was not pleasurable. I didn't really understand fully how much this had really affected my life. But as I grow older I become a little bit more aware. It's only recently that I've been able to identify myself as a survivor. It was easier to say I was a drug addict."

For a while, Rahema replaced one addiction with another and went into debt. "Every time I would go to a session I would have to come out and shop. I would buy myself something, 'cause I needed to do good things for myself. All that talk about me growing up, being in that house, feeling what it was like, all the anger and disappointment with my mother—it was hard."

The therapist suggested that she transfer her feelings to paper rather than her credit card and recommended that she read *The Courage to Heal Workbook*. Rahema found it extremely useful to write everything down. "I didn't think that I could ever have been abused by my brother. How could you love somebody who hurts you? It was hard for me to make that separation."

She says her therapist helped her through the conflicting feelings. "She said it doesn't mean you're crazy. It doesn't mean you're a bad person. She helped me begin to sort those feelings out, and work through them.

"And she would give me references of what a healthy relationship was. She'd say, 'People who love people don't do this.' She gave me an assignment once to go and watch some young kids in the schoolyard—about my age when I was abused—and I would just sit and watch them and then see how innocent they were. That helped me not be so conflicted about my feelings."

And Rahema remembered her own daughter, when she was about three, with redness in her genital area and white stuff oozing out of her vagina. Rahema had emerged from her haze of heroin to take her daughter to the hospital, where the doctor suggested that the child might have been abused. For some reason—she doesn't remember why—neither the police nor the city's child protection services personnel were called in to investigate. That night, she returned her daughter to her mother's chaotic home, and while she didn't point fingers, she accused everybody there of molesting her baby. She never linked her brother directly, but she knows he used to babysit. There were no more signs of abuse after that.

As Rahema grew stronger with the help of counseling, her sisters began to follow. Three are now off drugs and alcohol. Sober and drug-free, they now compare notes. Rahema now knows she wasn't the only prey in her family. "My sisters said, 'We believe you because this is what happened to us.' My oldest sister would tell about how the two oldest brothers would get her in the back of their room and hold her down and pull down her panties and get on top of her, and she would cry."

They told Rahema about how another sister kept the brothers away by threatening them with a knife. And they told about how their mother, who they believe is also a survivor, left the South at thirteen to get out of her own household. Rahema could see how she continued the pattern by escaping home at eighteen. "I used to be angry with them, but knowing about their abuse helped me see I wasn't alone. It helped us bond."

Rahema's mother refuses to talk about the abuse. "My mom would be like, 'How do you know?' You know. I would say because it's not normal for a kid to do all the things that I did to myself, and I would say because I remember some things. But she couldn't really deal." Rahema feels her mother has been so troubled by the loss of so many children that she cannot bear to see any of them in a negative light. "I think she was present physically, but I don't know how present she was emotionally," she says.

The brother who abused Rahema is one of those who died of AIDS, so she may never know the extent of the abuse. And at this point, that's okay, she says. What's most important is that she's off the drugs and making a life for herself and her family. An admirer of her work at the outreach agency suggested that she go back to school to get her degree. She first went to court and got her arrest warrants bundled together and did three years of probation and community service. She applied to a local college, and based on an essay about her life, she was awarded life-experience credits. She recently completed her master's in social work and is blazing trails in her department.

And she's learning to experience emotions, like anger, joy, happiness. She agreed to be interviewed for this book, she says, because she wants to encourage others to turn to therapy. "I still struggle with my inner child. It's hard because she's still very angry, very hurt. This has been so freeing, because abuse disconnected me. I didn't even have memories of being a child. It's like my life began in sixth grade. This has helped me be a parent to my kids, because that little girl was somewhere off in a corner and wasn't coming out."

Rahema joined a church and began to nurture her spirit, reading scripture and joining a Bible study group. With her new attitude and approach to life, she attracted a man who brought new energy into her life. Rahema's man, who is divorced and has an older child, specializes in holistic healing and practices bodywork. Rahema says he has taught her how to love. "I would say the first year I would cry every time he touched me. Sometimes I would cry so bad that we wouldn't even finish making love. He would just hold me and let me cry. I was a mess. It was like he was healing my spirit in a place it was broken. And I was so afraid to give myself to him because I had to learn that this was not about abuse, not money, not drugs. He didn't want me for my things. I am so thankful for him and what he has brought to my life." They recently had twin boys.

Rahema's daughter, the oldest of her four children, is now headed to college. Rahema has told her about the time she thinks her daughter was abused, and about her own memories of abuse. In one of her daughter's admissions essays, she was asked to tell about her role model. "She wrote about me," Rahema says. Then her eyes turn misty and she smiles. "That's priceless."

LORI'S STORY: DIGGING TO THE CORE

Few people really knew Lori, a popular hairstylist in Detroit. All they could really say was that she had a bad attitude and was one of the best in the city.

Sure, she took care of business: She was planning to open her own salon. But nearly everyone would agree she was "evil all the time," as Lori says. She knows that if she wasn't such a good stylist, her clients wouldn't have put up with her.

That negative attitude was Lori's shield, her protection against years of feeling used, unloved, and unaccepted. She used it with precision, keeping friends and family alike at a distance. It was also her protection against horrific reminders of abuse by her stepfather and father from age nine to nineteen. For most of her life, Lori, forty-one, kept those experiences locked away, buried under layers of depression, anger, and self-hate.

Behind her attitude, Lori was severely depressed. She would sit at home, scratching or cutting her arms and legs with razors; she would pull out her hair. That was how she silently, privately handled the pain of having been sexually abused. Lori managed to keep it all in check until New Year's Eve 2001, when she found herself staring at a pile of sleeping pills and a bottle of vodka.

How had it come to this? With the help of two therapists, Lori now knows why. "I always knew that something wasn't right," she says. "But I'd keep busy, immersing myself in work." But back then, on that cold night in December, she simply wanted to die.

It would have meant a bitter end to a sad and lonely life. Lori was raised in suburban Detroit, the eldest of three girls and a boy. Her mother worked a hospital job and attended college, and her stepfather was a school gym teacher. With busy schedules, the adults looked after themselves and Lori was left to look after the children.

In fact, Lori has spent most of her life taking care of everybody else. She describes her childhood as like Cinderella's: "always watching the kids, and always cleaning up." She also remembers feeling ugly. With her short, kinky hair and gangly body, she stood out among the younger, smaller, "cuter" kids with their long, wavy hair. At her Catholic school and at camp, she'd often hear, "Oh, your sister is so cute. What happened to you?" "Everybody used to tell me how ugly I was," she says.

"I don't remember much of growing up, don't remember playing with brother and sisters, don't remember games, or music, or anything else. I don't remember anything—except the chores, and the beatings if I disobeyed."

Then there was the terror. "Sometimes I'd be asleep. My stepfather would hit me and wake me up if I didn't do something right. A belt, switches, whatever. I just knew that he didn't like me." When she wasn't needed for chores, she says, she felt invisible.

Lori's stepfather was removed and reserved—he didn't talk with any of the kids. Her mother was distracted. In a house of six, Lori felt alone and unloved. She looked for signs that she mattered outside of the home, and found them in a neighborhood boy. That, she soon found, was a terrible mistake.

One day her stepfather caught nine-year-old Lori kissing the boy behind the garage. She knew she would be punished, but the beating she expected didn't come. Instead, he took her inside, into a bedroom. "He cleared off the bed and took my clothes off. Then he got on top of me, rubbin' and everything. He was trying to stick his penis in me, but he said something like, 'I'm not gonna put it all the way in, because that wouldn't be right.' So he would just be on me, sweatin'. Then he got up and went into the bathroom, and told me to go to my room."

She told no one, wanting to put her punishment behind her. But he began to abuse her regularly, often when everyone else was asleep. She reached out for help, telling the boy she had kissed. "All he said was, 'Nobody will believe you.'"

With that, Lori became sullen and withdrawn. At school, where she somehow kept up with the work, she began talking out and getting into fights. Lori couldn't find the words to tell her mother, she just hoped she would notice that something was different. But work and school and a husband and four kids vied for her attention.

The abuse became too much. One night Lori told her stepfather that she wanted him to die. "I told him I wasn't getting any sleep," she says. The next day, he died at work. "I felt like I'd killed him." She didn't speak for months. She was twelve years old.

Lori's biological father then came into her life, alerted by an aunt who thought that something was wrong with the girl. The aunt suspected that Lori's silence had something to do with her stepfather, and shared that hunch with Lori's father. Lori's mother thought it might do some good for her father to be in her life. Lori met her father for the first time after her stepfather died. And not long after, he began to molest her. "He said that since I did it before that I had to do it with him," Lori remembers. It started with touching, and soon it was rape.

"He would come to our house, saying he was coming to see my mother," she says. "Later, he would come in my room and close the door."

Lori tried to fight back, but she paid dearly. "When I would say no, bad things would happen to me," she says. "I would get beat. I would get punished. It was better not to say no." She threatened to tell, but he said nobody would believe her. She finally told her best friend, who told her sister, who told Lori's mother, who said, "You can't be going about telling lies. He's your father."

Lori shared the lessons she had learned in her young life: "I started to think, 'That's all you're good for.' I felt I was on my own. I learned that you don't go for help. You just pray and make it through." So when he came for sex, she would "blank out," or dissociate, as experts call it, so she would not have to endure the experience. The abuse continued for years, until she was finally old enough to move out.

Doing hair, Lori says, became her retreat and her anchor. "I would immerse myself in my school and work," she says, "so I didn't have much free time." Her fascination with hair began when her mother tried to give her a perm once, to "straighten out the kinks." It made her hair fall out, and she had to wear a wig for a while. She's been doing hair for a living since she was sixteen.

She managed to build a solid reputation and following, in spite of her attitude. She thought she had everything under control until about five years ago. "That's when life began chipping away at me," she says. First, a friend died in her arms. Then one friend lied and another stole some money she'd set aside for the new shop. One loss and two betrayals, all in a row.

Then, at thirty-eight, came perimenopause, with its irregular bleeding and night sweats. Hormone therapy brought sudden weight gain. Anxiety began to take hold and quickened Lori's spiral into depression. "It made me feel loss even more. I felt like I had lost something else that I didn't have control over. I didn't have control over my childhood, my teens. Then come to find out I cannot have children. I had lost my friend, lost trust in people, lost friends who I thought were in my corner.

"It all piled up. It was hard to speak to people. To touch people. When my nieces would come to visit, they would make me physically ill. I knew I was in trouble. I couldn't travel because I was afraid to fly. Sometimes I wouldn't go out other than to the salon. Then it had gotten to the point where I wouldn't go to work. Here I was, turning forty and thinking, 'You know I just wasted my whole life.' So I made a plan for the first of January. I said I would kill myself. The salon would be closed, so nobody would be looking for me. Friends would be away, so I figured that would be the perfect day. I got everything all ready."

But to her surprise, one friend knew her better than she thought. This was a friend in whom Lori had confided about her past and who believed her. This friend from time to time would casually suggest that Lori get professional help, but Lori declined each time. Somehow, this friend had a feeling about Lori on New Year's Eve.

"She called me from abroad," Lori says. "She had been calling me every day. She was telling me to go to church with a friend of hers. I kept saying, 'I don't want to go anywhere. I just want to stay home.'" Her friend pressed, until Lori snapped. "I started screaming at her that I just wanted to be left alone! I said I just want to go to sleep. It's always been so hard to say no, but right then I really meant no! So she got real quiet and said okay."

But that friend didn't turn away. She called another friend who lived nearby. By then Lori had started taking the pills and vodka. "Next thing she was ringing my bell. She came with a friend and they talked to me. They wouldn't leave. They cleaned my house and took care of me. The next day another friend came over to take me to church. And then another, and another. They wouldn't let me be by myself." When her friend returned to the States, she gave her the name of a therapist and told her she had to go. This time, Lori listened.

The psychologist tried to get Lori to talk about her past. In no time at all, they hit the core of her troubles. "She asked me something and it took me into a flashback. It was the worst thing I ever felt in my life. I started shaking and crying—I didn't understand it. And when I came out of it, I was exhausted." They tried again. "I flashed back to times when the sexual abuse was happening or I was getting beaten. I actually went back to that place. At one point I passed out."

The therapist knew Lori needed help to face such traumatic memories. She urged Lori to see a psychiatrist, who could prescribe medication. "She said I needed the medicine in order to even begin to talk about it. She thought it was too hard to go into these flashbacks and then come out." Lori was reluctant. But the therapist told her that she couldn't help her if she didn't take the medicine.

The psychiatrist told her she might have a chemical imbalance, possibly brought on by the trauma. He prescribed Paxil, a drug commonly used to treat depression and anxiety. At first, it made her terribly sleepy. But her body soon got used to it. It helped make Lori feel safe enough to talk about the abuse. And back in the psychologist's office, she was able to weather the flashbacks. They talked about how her experiences left her feeling unworthy, not good, unclean. About her fear of the word *no:* "When I would say no, then bad things would happen to me. I would get punished or people would get angry. It was better for me not to say no. I was tired of being hurt all the time."

Her psychologist, a sister, would push her "just so far," Lori says. "She knows how to talk to you in a way that it's not like you're in therapy. I can't deal with somebody saying, 'And how do you *feel?*' She can talk to me in a regular, everyday way. I don't feel like I'm in therapy. I just go in and have a little conversation."

And her psychiatrist, who is also Black, brings spirituality and philosophy into their conversations. "He talks about God and why we're here, how he's gonna get me to stop thinkin' about what I lost and start focusing on what I have in the future. I know you can't forget your past experiences. But what you can do is look at them differently. He's trying to give me another way of thinking and being." Lori has seen both for the last year.

When therapy turned to the subject of Lori's mother, her anxiety flared again. The psychologist invited Lori's mother in for a session. It seems that hearing about Lori's experience from a doctor helped convince her that her daughter was abused. Doubted for so many years, now Lori doesn't believe that her mother is sincere. "We're still working on this," she says. "I feel as if when I needed her, she wasn't there. So now why bother?"

Her treatment also had a surprising effect on the attitude that Lori had projected to the world. "I didn't feel really that much different, but when I went to work everybody said, 'Oh my God, Lori, you look great. You seem so happy.' So many people noticed a change. They were saying, 'You're so calm.'"

Lori, the girl who grew up taking care of everybody else, is learning how to take care of herself. One of the psychiatrist's "prescriptions" was regular exercise, something Lori has been slow to embrace. But she is working to change those things she can change in her life. "Goin' to the gym. Eating right. Taking more control over my work and how I work and when I work. Saying no." She is also learning the meaning of true friendship, and trust, whom to let go and whom to let in.

Lori's progress has been slow and tenuous. "It's still hard to get out of bed some days," she says. "But I know I've gotten better. I'm calmer. I can get on a plane and not be petrified. I can handle things that don't go right. I was slicing my wrists up, scratching myself till I bled. I don't do that now. It's easier to talk to people. It's easier to have the social contacts that I need in my business. At least I'm not takin' pills and drinking vodka all day."

She is still ambivalent about the medication. "I don't want to take it forever. I don't feel like it's really me. I'm used to being the person that people described as evil and ugly and serious. Now people want to be around me. Or people say positive things about me. It's hard to get used to. You've been one way for forty years and all of a sudden you're something else."

And then she stops for a moment, and as if realizing how much work she has to do, she sighs. "If I stopped taking it, tomorrow I would be right back where I was."

SHANTEL'S STORY: A HEALER HELPS HERSELF

Shantel, a thirty-eight-year-old Boston social worker, was a perfectionist and a "control freak," upsetting her son and driving her husband crazy. Their marital relationship had long ago lost its intimacy. She was also carrying heavy secrets, which in spite of her professional experience, she would have just as soon kept to herself.

Shantel had one foot out of her nearly eighteen-year marriage. And she was afraid of where the next step might lead. Her husband, Tony, had turned away and seemed to be headed toward other women. They agreed to see a therapist.

Counseling was where Shantel and Tony would finally discuss her years of abuse by her mother's boyfriend—from when she was thirteen until she left for college. This was the man whom Tony had befriended as a father-in-law. The man who had walked Shantel down the aisle. The man whom her mother had gone to the grave loving. Whom her grandmother—the closest thing Shantel had to a mother since her own had died—embraced as a son. How could so many lives become so twisted around such an ugly past?

Shantel's answer: fear, loss, loneliness, and deep, deep shame.

By the time Nate, her mother's boyfriend, came along, Shantel was already familiar with violation and the secrecy that often surrounds it. She was raped at nine. It was an eighteen-year-old who lived up the street. Like most girls in the neighborhood, she remembers, she had a crush on him. She was on an errand for a pack of cigarettes at the store when she passed a bunch of boys. To her delight, the one she liked peeled off to walk with her. She couldn't believe her luck. "Somebody likes me," she remembers thinking. He led her to the rooftop of a nearby building. There, behind a giant neon fast-food sign, he forced her to the ground. When he was done, he left without a word.

She never told anyone what happened up there on the roof, afraid that she would get in trouble. Shantel was raised by her mother, a grandmother, her great-grandmother, and an aunt. In this house full of women the rules were strict for the only child: "You respected your elders, and you did not talk back," she says. Physical discipline was the norm. Her mother was a nurse, and Shantel can recall their candid, sometimes nurturing talks. "I had gotten my period, and she told me about using tampons," she says. They talked about sex. "She'd say, 'I know you have feelings, but you need to be more mature before you go out and engage in that kind of activity.'"

Even so, Shantel recalls, she couldn't bring up the rape. "I would get tore up!" she says. She could already hear her grandmother repeating what she often told her mom: "You need to keep a better watch on Shantel—I'm not her babysitter."

When Nate, her mother's boyfriend, started abusing her, she reasoned to herself that if she had kept that earlier secret, she could keep another.

Shantel was thirteen when her mother started seeing Nate. He was somebody her mother had met at the hospital. Shantel remembers being angry that her mother was being taken away by some strange man. About a year after they got together, Shantel and her mother moved into his place. It wasn't so bad, Shantel thought, because he bought her everything she wanted. But then he began to do things like leave the bathroom covered only by a washcloth. She mentioned her unease to her mother, saying, "I don't like the way he kisses. It's a little too long. He wants to hug a little too tight." Her mother asked him to stop.

Nate simply waited until Shantel's mother left for work. "He would kiss me and feel me up all over," she says. Shantel told her mother again, and the three of them sat down to talk about it. His response to her mother, Shantel remembers, was this: "You have to understand, I love you, but I also love her." Shantel and her mother moved out.

But her mother continued to see him. Shantel says her mother posted a number to a child abuse hotline on the refrigerator. "I think she thought if we no longer lived together then it would stop," she says. It didn't.

Over the next few years, she says, "He would come over when my mother was at work, kissing, fondling, and digitally penetrating me. Eventually I became used to it and, thinking I was taking the upper hand, I told myself I would allow it to occur if I could get money to keep quiet. If I needed a new coat he'd buy it. If Mama said, 'We can't afford it,' he'd say, 'Well, here, let her get it.' At Christmastime, it was overboard."

Looking back, Shantel can see how she was prepared for abuse, a process experts call grooming. Meanwhile, Nate became a trusted member of the extended family.

When she left for college, Shantel was ready to tell her mother about the abuse. But doctors found cancer in her mother, and the disease quickly took its toll. Shantel kept quiet. "She had so much to deal with," she says.

Shantel chose a local college to be near home. She stayed away from Nate, except when she needed money. "I began to reason, 'So what if I let him kiss me? That's all it was.' I thought I had control of the situation. I wouldn't let him near me unless I was getting something in return, and that was mostly money. My mother couldn't afford school. I had loans up the wazoo. So if I needed $50 he could get what he wanted. If he wanted to kiss me, to fondle me, I'd let him. I was really disgusted with myself."

She met Tony her freshman year. He was one of a long line of men. "I entered into many sexual liaisons because I thought that was what men wanted, and that was my best asset. I figured if this is what men think of me, then this is what I'm going to be. Thank God I never got pregnant, never contracted a disease. But I put myself in dangerous situations."

Tony proposed just before her mother died. "So she went to her grave not knowing what happened," Shantel says. She remembers being angry, sad, and bitter. "I thought, how *dare* she leave me here to deal with these issues!" They married after they graduated. Tony, who is now a minister, is a year older than Shantel. And as she sees it, he's also her opposite. "He's laid back, very quiet, conservative," she says. "I'm the outgoing one, the bubbly type." One of the few things they have in common is their struggle to communicate.

I ask Shantel what made her marry a man so different, and at such a young age. She sighs. "Let's just put it this way: I don't want to say a way out. But what I saw was someone who fell in love with me, who wanted to take care of me. And I think that's what I needed. My mother had died. I was very, very needy. And he was the first person who really saw me for me." She stops and corrects herself. "But he did not see all of me. He only saw what I was willing to show."

When Tony and Shantel had their son, Nate sent a card saying he had hoped the boy would be his. Tony saw it and became furious. He thought

Shantel was having an affair. Shantel finally had to tell him about the abuse.

Tony wanted to kill Nate. He was angry and hurt. He kept asking why. Why had she let Tony grow to like him? Why had she let him walk her down the aisle? She knew her answers rang hollow. She had put up the front for years, she said, and she was afraid. "I was worried about what people would think. Everybody loved Nate—my grandmother loved him."

Tony wanted to confront Nate, but Shantel said no. "This was my issue, and I had to handle it. It had nothing to do with him." Tony backed off.

And so life went on, with the secret out and the wounds open. The revelation weighed on their relationship. Shantel became angry and controlling, and Tony became withdrawn. They talked less and less, and intimacy and sex became rare. Then she learned of his adventures with an online dating service and found a suggestive note from him to a family friend. Shantel and Tony knew they had to try to save their marriage. So they agreed to see a counselor.

At first, Tony insisted on a pastoral counselor, and Shantel refused. She considered herself a spiritual person, but as a mental health professional, she wanted someone with expertise in trauma and family dynamics and anger. Eventually Tony agreed to see a professional as long as it wasn't someone Shantel knew, and Shantel contacted her insurance company for a referral. They were sent to a White male psychologist. After a few meetings, Shantel said, they became quite comfortable with him.

The couple started with what was true. "I know he loves me, I know he's very committed to me. And he just wants to be heard," Shantel says.

Then they moved to the abuse. Tony talked about his frustration, about not being able to help, and about her need to control. She didn't like having her issues aired in the open, but she had to admit her husband was right. "I realized, I am letting all of this dictate who I am and who I'm going to be. It got to the point that when my husband did the dishes and put something where it didn't belong, you could hear me yelling, 'I don't know *why* people don't put things back where they belong!' If he made the bed, I would unmake it and make it again because he didn't use hospital corners. It was driving him crazy."

With the therapist's help, Shantel came to see how her need to control everything stemmed from being abused. "I need to have control, because I didn't have control growing up," she told her husband. The psychologist talked about the long-term effects of abuse, helping her husband see that Shantel's responses to her experience were common.

Their troubles were also affecting their son, and it started to show at school. One day he simply asked his parents if they were getting a divorce. "We said no, we were not getting a divorce, but we were going to a marriage counselor," she says. "I said, 'Sometimes you need a third person to help figure things out.' That helped put him at ease."

Marriage counseling led Shantel to take a hard look at herself. "I spent so much time blaming Tony. I had to realize I was partly responsible for how he was acting. He just doesn't know what he's going to face when he comes home. Am I going to be sweet and loving, or am I going to be a bitch on wheels?"

She began to see a therapist on her own. "I found myself increasingly dealing with the effects of the abuse. The promiscuity, the low self-esteem, my weight—all of that was finally out. It wasn't consuming me, but it was there." She has learned to manage her anger, to be mindful of her tendencies to be controlling. "It works at the job. But at home, I've learned to let things go."

And as for Nate, she relied on faith. "I cast that up to God," she says. "I said, 'You deal with that. It no longer has a hold on my life.'" As a way of closing that ugly chapter of her life, Shantel calculated how much money she had taken from Nate over the years, and she sent him a check for that amount. He has never cashed it. Shantel wasn't fazed by his lack of response. It was more important that she resolve her past.

Does she still have issues? "This doesn't mean I won't still get angry, but I'm not going to hold on to that anger anymore. I refuse to let anybody destroy my peace. Am I 100 percent healed? No, but I am on my way."

Where do things stand with Tony? It's hard to tell. "He's supportive, but he's kind of backed away. I know it had an impact on our sex life. Sexually, I don't think we were overly compatible to begin with. But it was much more active before I told him. It's less frequent, and there's not much touching or cuddling."

Slowly, they're learning to communicate, and they're working on intimacy. "It used to be that he wouldn't say anything; he would just let things fester. Now he's able to check in. I like that. And if I don't want to talk about it, he doesn't get upset. I think he needs to understand that if I want to be intimate, it doesn't necessarily mean in the physical sense. It could just be cuddling, watching a movie, without having to put out.

"But at the same time, when I ask and he says, 'No, maybe tomorrow,' I can't assume he must be with somebody else. It's something we're still working on."

Shantel has learned how she could use her experience for good. She works with children who have been abused and neglected, and with juveniles who have committed sexual offenses. Before that, she investigated sex abuse in families. "I believe in divine order," she says. "I'd like to think I was placed here for a reason."

She's working on a second master's degree—in criminal justice—and plans to work with sexual abusers. "Some say they would never want to deal with a perpetrator," she says, "but to work with either population you have to know about the other. And in working with offenders, as a survivor, I can help them understand the impact their crimes have had on that child. So I'm trying to help them break that cycle."

Shantel shares the story of one young client, a foster child. "Her mother was killed and she suffered horrendous abuse from her natural family and her foster family," she says. "All the siblings were made to engage in sexual activity with one another. It was extreme. Carving words into herself. Trying to set her bed on fire. She ended up with multiple personalities. Her case workers kept changing, because they couldn't handle her. I stayed with her, I listened to her. She was one of the first kids I disclosed to. I said, 'I know what you're going through, 'cause I've been where you've been. I want to let you know that you can get over this.'

"I pushed for her to get specialized treatment. She's now out of the system. She has her own apartment, a job, and she's involved in her church. She e-mails me every month. Once when I went to visit, we drove to see her therapist. And she told me, 'I know you never put yourself in this role, but I want to thank you for being a mom.' It was the first time she got that nurturing. And she said, 'Someday I want to be like you. I want to be able to say that this is my history, not my future.' And that makes it worthwhile."

COMMON GROUND

Rahema, Lori, and Shantel each turned to talk therapy as a way to heal. While their circumstances differed, they shared problems common among many survivors:

- Anger
- Emotional distance
- Risky or destructive behavior

- Troubled relationships with partners or other family members
- Trouble developing or maintaining intimate relationships
- Struggles with issues of trust

But throughout their common problems runs a common thread: hope. Their haunting stories show that we can never be too far gone to heal. With the guidance of trained professionals, each woman found a way to acknowledge her past, understand its effects, and make concrete steps toward improving her life. For some survivors, like Tracey, who turned to dance, or Karen, who turned to books, alternative approaches prove to be extremely helpful as well. In the next chapter I will explore ways to help children heal.

HELP YOURSELF

African-Centered Healing

Rhonda Wells-Wilbon, who teaches social work at Morgan State University in Baltimore, is a sexual abuse survivor. She had spent years in and out of traditional counseling before she met an African-centered therapist who changed the way she approached healing.

The therapist helped her build a foundation of "a new knowledge base and new skills," says Wells-Wilbon, "starting with *reconciliation*, an important African value, which means simply the act of restoring and making harmonious." Knowing the importance of reconciliation, she says, "I realized that I had to tell my parents how angry I had been all those years and that I forgave them for not knowing. It was not until I had some crucial conversations with them about the abuse and my feelings that I was able to reconcile how such a terrible thing happened to me. It was not until then that I felt able to move from being a victim."

Wells-Wilbon uses this approach not just for herself but also to teach her students how to counsel Black clients in a way that acknowledges and validates our history, customs, and traditions, as well as our cultural perspective on the world.

What does it mean to be African-centered? It is simply using Africa "as a geographical and cultural starting point for the study of African people," she says, as opposed to viewing them through a Eurocentric lens.

An African-centered approach can help us rediscover ways of healing that are rooted in the traditions of our ancestors. Among those traditions is the ancient Egyptian principle of Ma'at. Estimated to have been written two thousand years before the Ten Commandments, Ma'at is considered a foundation of natural and social order and unity and is widely accepted among many scholars of Black psychology. Ma'at is characterized by seven cardinal virtues, as described in *The Psychology of Blacks: An African Centered Perspective,* which are considered a "code of conduct and a standard of aspiration."[17] When practiced, the seven virtues of Ma'at are said to provide stability amid chaos and dysfunction:

- Truth (openness)—sincerity in speech, behavior, and character that is in accord with fact
- Justice—principle of just and right action where fairness and equality reign
- Righteousness/propriety (integrity)—acting in accord with divine or moral law
- Harmony (peace, beauty, grace)—proper arrangement or alignment of things so they function together
- Order (civility, formality)—the natural and harmonious arrangement of things that helps define one's purpose
- Balance—stability produced by an even distribution of elements
- Reciprocity (compassion, patience)—giving of oneself, sharing

I asked Wells-Wilbon to adapt these ancient principles to modern-day living for survivors of child sexual abuse. She provided what she calls the Aya Model for healing, named after *aya,* the Andinkra symbol for the hardy fern plant that flourishes in harsh and difficult terrain. Her Aya Model encourages us to perform rituals—routines connected with a solemn, sacred, or important event. In his writings, the African scholar Malidoma Somé explains how rituals can help solve problems when words alone will not do. But for rituals to work, he writes, we must be receptive to their healing power: "Success in a ritual is proportional to the level of surrender that one can achieve. Because ritual is about change, its success depends on how much change, and what change, if any, we are willing to invite."[18] Wells-Wilbon shares the following African-centered rituals and practices for easing the trauma, sorrow, and sense of loss that stems from sexual abuse.

Rhonda Wells-Wilbon's Aya Model: Ten Steps Toward Healing

1. **Go natural.** Wear your hair in a style that celebrates its natural texture, Wells-Wilbon recommends. Wear natural fibers. Eat live foods like fresh fruits and vegetables. Remove the barriers between you and nature as you move closer to your own center. As Somé writes: "Every tree, plant, hill, mountain, rock and each thing that was here before us

emanates or vibrates at a subtle energy that has healing power whether we know it or not. So if something in us must change, spending time in nature provides a good beginning."[19]

2. **Form circles.** Circles represent the endless cycles of life, death, and rebirth. Circles eliminate the need for hierarchical structure in rela- tionships. Think of the exchanges that take place within sister circles and prayer circles. When she teaches, Wells-Wilbon says, "I always ask that people sit in a circle, and I always join that circle as a teacher—and a student."

3. **Incorporate water.** Water is a life force that can bring serenity and focus. Before a child is born, Wells-Wilbon reminds us, she lives in the water of her mother's womb. The first water ritual she incorporated into her life was libation, a call to the ancestors, inviting them to be present. A libation is usually conducted by pouring water into a living plant while calling names of ancestors, she explains. A healing bath can become a ritual: Scent it with rosemary or lavender oil, surround it with candles or incense, and complement it with a favorite meditation CD. Wells-Wilbon also practices a special cleansing ritual during gath- erings and in trainings. In it, each person gets an opportunity to cleanse his or her hands and soul while reciting, "Just as my ancestors cleansed themselves in the rivers of the Nile, today I cleanse myself of [name the thing that you want to be rid of]."

4. **Incorporate fire.** Fire opens the door to the spirit world, notes Malidoma Somé. As we walk the earth, he says, we are warmed by the heat of the ancestors coming from the underworld below us. Wells- Wilbon's fire rituals include burning candles throughout her home and office and using her fireplace regularly in the cold seasons. Occasionally she writes on little pieces of paper the things she wants out of her life, and she burns them in a glass bowl or aluminum tin.

5. **Practice aromatherapy.** Noting that our ancestors used incense as a part of their spiritual rituals, Wells-Wilbon continues the practice at home. She burns incense and oils like lavender, which is known for its calming effect. And you can easily find scented candles and potpourri. At the office, she uses scented plug-in air fresheners. She also makes a point to stop and enjoy the scents of nature, such as the ocean, a rose, or the burning of wood.

6. **Speak your truth.** Speaking truth to power is essential to healthy liv-

ing. Wells-Wilbon urges: "Tell your own story in your own words, and in your own time. It is only then that real healing can begin." This can also mean learning the truth about Africa and an African-centered view. "I have found that knowledge of African values is a critical building block of my foundation for healing," she says.

7. **Practice reciprocity.** Sharing in a way that helps others is an important part of your own healing. This is one reason many survivors become healers themselves. After graduating from college, Wells-Wilbon worked at a crisis hotline for a sexual assault center. Later she led a shelter program for abused women and their children. "Whenever appropriate, I share my experiences so that others get the courage to tell their own stories," she says. "Sharing is an action that opens a path for others to take to heal."

8. **Find order.** Harmony and balance—the ultimate goals of a healthy life—require order. This means getting rid of clutter, being organized, making lists, keeping a schedule, and more. You may not be good at all of these all the time, Wells-Wilbon says, but moving toward order can create positive energy in your life.

9. **Know who you are.** We all have the power to define ourselves from our own perspective and view of the world. This power, also known by the Kwanzaa principle Kujichagulia, or self determination, "Is especially dear to a people who for generations did not even own their bodies," Wells-Wilbon says. This power is not something we need to claim; it already resides within each of us. And in the face of the many nonaffirming or offensive messages that we so often receive, it is enormously empowering to be able to define who you are and what you will be. "There are many ways to define yourself by way of your ancestry," Wells-Wilbon says, "whether it is claiming an African name or wearing African clothing or accents or simply knowing your heritage and culture."

10. **Find your purpose.** If you start with the premise that each of us has a divine reason for being on this earth, Wells-Wilbon says, it is our responsibility to determine why. "Recognize what makes you you—and not just your gifts and talents," she says, "but also your experiences and unique perspective." Knowing these things, she says, ask yourself, "Am I using all that I am in a way that benefits me, my family, and my community?" If the answer is no, find out how you can. Ask friends, family, counselors, and spiritual advisers for guidance. Know that your

sense of purpose will change as you have new experiences, grow wiser, and gain more insight. "Being African-centered has helped give me clarity on my life's purpose," she says. "I know I was abused because someone else's life was so out of balance that they were troubled and confused. I also know that as a professional social worker, I've found my true purpose, which is helping others who may not otherwise have the opportunity to heal."

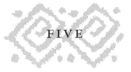

FIVE

Protecting and Saving Our Children

*I honestly believed that what was occurring between my father and me
was what occurred between all fathers and daughters.
I felt connected and special with my dad.*

—CAROL, who was abused by her father for six years

PARENTING IS THE MOST IMPORTANT CALLING YOU WILL EVER HAVE. You are charged with loving and nurturing a human being—a living, breathing entity who does not come with instructions. The day-to-day work of rearing a child can be daunting in and of itself. But most of us also have jobs, with their own time-and-energy-consuming issues and drama. Then there are responsibilities to our partners and our church, and other community-building obligations that demand our attention. In our effort to keep all the commitments in the air, we sometimes lose sight of the most important: our children. But when our children are number one, all other priorities fall into place.

It wasn't until I had my son seven years ago—until I held him in my hands—that I fully appreciated how dependent children are on those who take care of them. And when it was time for me to return to work and leave my baby with a sitter, I was terrified. "How could I trust him with a stranger?" I agonized. I would call home several times a day, make surprise visits to pick up something I'd "forgotten," and spy on them regularly at the playground until I felt my son was secure.

What enormous faith we parents must have to put our children in some-

Fast Facts

- Sixty-seven percent of all victims of sexual assault reported to police were under the age of eighteen; one in every seven victims—14 percent—was under age six.[1]
- Strangers were offenders in just 3 percent of assaults against children six and under and in 5 percent of assaults of children six to eleven.[2]
- In one study, the average age that parents gave as most appropriate for them to talk to their children about sexual abuse was 9.1 years.[3] Statistics show that children are more vulnerable to sexual abuse starting at age eight.[4] And among children under twelve, four-year-olds are at greatest risk of being a victim of assault.[5]
- Up to 66 percent of pregnant teens report histories of sexual abuse.[6]
- In a study of college students, those women at higher risk of sexual abuse were the ones who said they were not close to their mothers or received little affection from their mothers or fathers.[7]

one else's charge. If that person is not a relative or family friend, we try to get a sense of their character through interviews and references. Rightly so, we carefully monitor their actions and interactions for even the slightest signs to confirm our worst fears. But if the caregiver is already under our umbrella of friend and family, then we are more likely to give them the benefit of doubt than scrutiny. That's because we're relying on them to hold up their end of the unspoken family trust.

Irma and Allen could not bring themselves to believe that their daughter, Maya, was abused by Maya's grandfather (Chapter 3). The benefit of doubt came all too easily, and at their daughter's expense. "I never saw anything that would make me think he could do something like that," Irma said. "And I kept saying, 'Oh, Maya, it must be a bad dream.'" Irma and Allen, like many of us would, assumed that Maya's grandfather would feel the same obligation to protect her that they did because of the family trust. Unfortunately, this is a common assumption. Without evidence, many parents will even ignore their own suspicions. The problem is that for all too many children, there is no definitive evidence.

So who will protect our children from sexual abuse? The adults in their lives must take responsibility. Many of us are clearly safety-conscious: We strap our kids in car seats and seat belts, we hold their hands when they cross the street, we cushion them in protective gear when they ride bikes. We ingrain in them the rules we learned to navigate life's dangers: don't run with sharp objects; call 911 when someone is hurt; stop, drop, and roll in case clothing catches fire. We can't assume that they will know to look out for a predator when they don't even know what one is. We need to become proactive and add sexual abuse safety to their list of precautions. We need to talk with them, encourage them to talk with us, and then *listen to them*. And we need to teach them to think critically, to trust their feelings, and to speak up if they are made to feel uncomfortable. But before we focus on ways to protect our children, let's first look at what we're protecting them from.

WHAT WE'RE UP AGAINST

You can't spot abusers just by looking at them or by watching how they interact with children. They can be anybody: a relative, a neighbor, a community leader, a professional. They try to appear trustworthy. They are methodical, conniving, and relentless. They have no problem smiling in your face and can even have sex with you while they plot to get at your kids.[8] They will work to convince children that they should be open to sexual advances or that they like being violated. As a part of their sickness, many cannot comprehend that their actions are harmful, or that the rules and laws that govern the rest of society apply to them. Their focus is on their own need for emotional or sexual gratification. Sexual abusers will not give up until they succeed in meeting that need, and once successful, many will continue until they are forced to stop. Child sexual abuse has been likened to an addiction. Research proves that once a victim shows resistance or grows up or moves out, a sexual abuser will often move on to the next child.

There is not yet a proven way to eliminate sexually abusive behavior, and as a society, our methods for responding to abuse and violence against children in general are relatively new. In many communities, children, as women once were, are still considered property. Consider this: The Child Abuse Prevention and Treatment Act (CAPTA), the first key federal legislation addressing child abuse and neglect in the United States, was enacted only in 1974.[9]

Today, every state has a mandatory reporting law, which requires all professionals who work with children (like doctors, teachers, and social workers) to report suspicions of sexual abuse to child protective services agencies or the police.

One widely popular recent response to sexual abuse was Megan's Law, named after Megan Kanka, a seven-year-old New Jersey girl who was raped and killed by a convicted child molester who had moved across the street from her family without their knowledge. Under the federal statute, which was established in 1996, each state must register convicted sex offenders and make information about them available to the public. On the Web, the FBI coordinates a Sex Offender Registry, a national database with links to information provided by the states (http://www.fbi.gov/hq/cid/cac/states.htm).

How helpful the law and the registries have been is debatable, given that most child sex offenders are already known and trusted by their victims, and only about one in ten children reports abuse.[10] But what is clear is that these kinds of measures do not stop abuse. In fact, they are effective only *after* abuse occurs. Meanwhile, society's reluctance to address the severity of the problem provides just the cloak of silence and secrecy that enables abusers to operate below the radar.

What motivates sexual abusers? The answer is rarely as simple as sexual desire. Theories abound on their emotional and psychological makeup: that they lack social skills, they're immature, repressed, perverse, senile, sexually frustrated, narcissistic, that they were victimized themselves as children, and on and on. Bottom line: Abusers act on an urge to feel powerful. That power can be physical, through force, but it also can be emotional or psychological, through intimidation, lies, and tricks. With age, size, and experience over their prey, sexual abusers have the obvious advantage. Once they are intent on abusing a child and they encounter no obstacles, they will find a way to do so. According to researcher David Finkelhor, these four preconditions must exist for abuse to occur:[11]

1. *There is a person who seeks a child out for sexual relations.* For this person, relating to the child satisfies some emotional or sexual need.
2. *The person overcomes internal inhibitions against abusing.* Abusers will often cite alcohol or drugs, which lower inhibitions, as the cause of their actions. But, as Finkelhor notes, the desire to act is present first; the substances make it easier to act on the desire. Mental illness has also been cited as a factor in blocking inhibitions.
3. *The person overcomes external obstacles or prohibitions against abusing.* A child who lacks appropriate supervision, is socially isolated within the family, lives in a home with unusual sleeping or rooming conditions, or in which family dynamics are chaotic, could be seen as fair game.

4. *The person overcomes or undermines resistance by the child.* Abusers are drawn to children who are emotionally insecure or deprived. Some take advantage by building trust with the child. They are unlikely to face challenges if the child is ignorant about abuse. In some cases, they simply use force to get their way.

The reality of Finkelhor's preconditions is that parents do not have the luxury of thinking that "this won't happen to my kid" or fearing that informing their children about sexual abuse will frighten or harm them in some way. For their own protection, children from a very young age need to know what the term *sexual abuse* means, what actions and behaviors constitute sexual abuse, and what they can and should do if someone tries to abuse them. We will explore some good ways to inform children without scaring them.

When abuse is disclosed, parents can get caught up in blaming themselves or their child, and let blame and embarrassment keep them from acknowledging and responding in a way that protects and helps the child. For adults who have been abused themselves, discovering that a child has been victimized can be paralyzing because it conjures up all the old trauma, along with its feelings of fear, self-blame, and helplessness. But how you respond to a child's disclosure of abuse can make all the difference in how the child begins to heal. We will also explore the best ways to do that.

A sexually victimized child will go to great lengths to mask any signs of the source of her guilt and shame, even while she's displaying symptoms of abuse by "acting out." Often, out of obligation to the abuser, a child may help to keep the secret hidden. How does this happen? Children want to be loved and are eager to please, and abusers know how to take advantage of them.

CAROL'S STORY: HOW CHILDREN ARE EASY PREY

Carol, thirty-six, a San Francisco marketing director, was abused by her father from age three to age nine. Early on, she says, "I honestly believed that what was occurring between my father and me was what occurred between all fathers and daughters. In my child's mind, I felt connected and special with my dad."

Carol grew up with her parents and older brother in nearby Oakland. From all appearances, hers was a typical striving family: With two parents earning income, Carol and her brother attended private schools and after-school activities, and they each got cars when they were old enough to drive. Inside Carol's home, however, was a world the neighbors would have never suspected. "It was rather innocent at first, not violent or intimidating," she says, describing the abuse. "There was never a threat, no 'I'm gonna hurt someone or myself or you.' It was just our secret."

Their secret started one night when Carol tiptoed out to the sunroom, where her father, a carpenter with sporadic work, was sleeping off his regular drinking binge. He was a "raging weekend alcoholic" who demanded respect in his home or else, Carol says. When he felt he wasn't getting it, he would physically and verbally abuse Carol's mother and brother, who was six years older. "I actually felt sorry for him," she says of her father. "He seemed so unhappy and angry. Even as a little girl, I sensed his troubles and wanted to make him feel better. I felt like if I loved him enough, he wouldn't do the bad things to my mother or brother." When three-year-old Carol went to the sunroom to tell her daddy that she loved him that night, he coaxed her into joining him on the floor.

That secret was easy to keep because Carol didn't know that what was happening was wrong, and she didn't talk much with her mother, who worked odd hours as a hospital clerk. "We didn't have the normal mother-daughter relationship," she said. "She went to all the parent-teacher conferences and the like, but there was no bond. We didn't talk about anything too deep. We never had the sex talk. I didn't feel I could really ask my mother questions about my maturing body, my thoughts, or even my future. That feeling continues today." Carol turned to her few friends and their mothers for guidance through puberty.

While her father lashed out at her brother and mother, he wouldn't hit Carol. She recalls only one spanking as a child, and little physical affection that wasn't sexual. But her father shared with her an intimacy meant for full-grown women. "It progressed from touching and fondling to kissing, he and I being naked, simulation of intercourse and, finally, an attempt at penetration," she says. "I don't remember actual penetration, but I do recall excruciating pain in the genital area. I recall my father's penis being extremely close to my face, and I hate to think or remember why. A few years ago I began to vividly remember smells, movements, and positions. I have memories of being in my parents' bed when my mother wasn't home."

Carol longed to have her father's attention when he wasn't furious with the world and taking it out on the family. And she hungered for his approval. So when Daddy did turn to her, she was cooperative. Looking back with the help of years of therapy, she sees how she was easy prey: "Like offering water to a person in a desert who is dying of thirst, I was offered intimacy, special privilege, and rewards."

Carol, who is now working toward a doctorate in clinical psychology, described the confusing mix of emotions and reactions that children can have when lured into a sexual relationship with someone who is supposed to protect them. "Children are taught to obey and accept the behaviors of their parents or elders; we couldn't question them, even if it seemed odd," she says. "Children also come into this world in great need of nurturing, affection, and touch. And little kids will respond to sexual touch. To some degree it's pleasurable." In Carol's mind, she distinguished between the abuse her father inflicted on her mother and brother and the abuse he inflicted on her. "I thought this was my father and he wouldn't do anything to hurt me, although he was violent in other ways. But the sexual abuse never seemed to be violent. It seemed more nurturing."

AN ABUSER'S TRICKS AND TOOLS

From the beginning, Carol's father made her pliable and compliant. He began early and his advances were subtle, so much so that she found her sexual relationship "nurturing." His was one of many methods that abusers use. As we've seen in previous chapters, abusers use several different tactics and typically monitor their victims' reactions and adjust their approach accordingly.[12] Here are the tools of their trade.

Grooming or Conditioning

This is one of the most common approaches. The abuser starts by working to gain the child's trust, as well as the family's trust. He may show an intense interest in the child, often to the exclusion of other children. Offers to babysit, play alone with the child, take the child for treats, or give the child presents should all be regarded with suspicion. "If some adult is showing your child more attention than you do, that's cause for alarm," says Ronda Hicks, a former counselor with the Coalition on Child Abuse and Neglect in suburban New York City. The abuser tries to bond with the child in a nonsexual way, perhaps by doing good deeds or confiding a personal or embarrassing story. That's a first secret that they share. If she's of an age where she's self-conscious or awkward about her body and her peers, he may tell her she's beautiful and easy to talk to. The goal is to isolate the child and make her feel important and connected. The abuser will be patient; this process could take days or even years. Once he knows that he has the child's trust, he will begin to sexualize the relationship. There is no typical order for it to occur, but it often progresses in a way that Carol experienced. An abuser may start by walking from room to room naked, leaving the door open while in the bathroom. He may share images from pornographic magazines or Web sites. He may make sexual comments about her body or the way she dresses, or tell stories and jokes not fit even for adult company. Then comes a touch, a kiss on the mouth, nudity, full-body contact, and attempts at intercourse or actual intercourse. He may stimulate the child's genitals and coax the child to stimulate his, by hand or mouth. Each new act builds upon a previous violation of the child, which is built upon the foundation of trust that the abuser worked so diligently to establish. Remember, no threat or physical force is necessary when the abuser has succeeded in cultivating trust and secrecy. The abuser may "reward" the child with gifts or money, making her feel as if she is a willing participant if she accepts. Sixteen-year-old Connie would keep the money that her mother's boyfriend slipped under her bedroom door (Chapter 2), and even though she never saw the man outside of her mother's presence, she knew there was a sexual nature to his gifts. Today she acknowledges the shame she felt, as she put it, for trying to take her mother's man. Actually, her mother's man was grooming her for sex.

Playing Games

For some abusers, games are their grooming process. Tickling and wrestling enable them to casually fondle the child, blurring the lines between appropriate and inappropriate touch. With games like these, an abuser has an easy out if the child expresses discomfort or tells someone what's happened. Here he can feign ignorance and present the violation as a "misunderstanding" or an accidental slip of the hand. Some games are more intricate, such as show-and-tell, truth or dare, or mimicking. The goal is to create a diversion for sexual behavior to occur before a child realizes what is happening, as Douglas Pryor writes in *Unspeakable Acts: Why Men Sexually Abuse Children,* a book based on in-depth interviews with thirty abusers: "Use of a game or play strategy, in general, allowed offenders to instigate sex in an apparently less threatening and non-forceful way, in a manner that to their victims probably appeared to involve an element of fun."[13]

Sneaking and Surprising

Some abusers violate children when they think the children aren't aware of it. For instance, Maya's grandfather (Chapter 3) would enter her bedroom and touch her while he thought she was sleeping. Again, abusers want to get to the child before she realizes and can react. The child may pretend to be asleep to avoid confrontation, or toss and turn to make an abuser think she's waking up. This approach also provides cover for abusers. Maya's mother continuously suggested that Maya must have dreamed up the abuse by her grandfather. Sneaking has many forms. One woman wrote to me, "I've caught my husband 'watching' my teenage daughter sleeping. Should I be worried?" The answer is, yes, absolutely. For some abusers, peeping is the first step toward a sexual encounter.

Seeking Sympathy and Enlisting Help

When Darlene's brother-in-law (Chapter 1) sought her help for his "problem"—that his wife was too pregnant for sex—eleven-year-old Darlene felt obliged to help. Similarly, abusers have been known to groom children by sharing "problems" and other details from their sex lives with adult partners, as if the children themselves were adults.[14]

Seduction

Preying on a child's natural need for affection, an abuser will use cuddling as an opportunity to cross the line to sexual touching. Stephanie's father began to touch her as she sat in his lap while watching TV (Chapter 2). Children may be too startled by the advance or too intimidated or confused or afraid to resist. Or they may not know that they should or can say or do anything to stop it. An abuser will typically test a victim after each new, more invasive violation, checking for her reaction. If he finds no resistance, he will take that as a sign that she's enjoying it or that his seduction is working, and he will proceed.[15]

On the other hand, some offenders might justify their actions by saying that the child seduced them. As several survivors acknowledged, children can feel pleasure during abuse, much to their shame. But there is nothing to feel shameful about, as the clinical psychologist Dorothy Cunningham reminded us when referring to the confusion of Kim, who spoke of being titillated and repulsed at the same time when she anticipated having sex with her stepfather (Chapter 2): "You can be terrified and confused but still have an orgasm," Cunningham says. "Her body did what bodies are supposed to do—it responded to touch. That's how bodies are made." Sexual offenders will take a child's confusion and silence to mean that they are enjoying the abuse and want it to continue.

But even if an offender says he was seduced, most experts agree that children are incapable of consenting to sex with adults because they don't truly know what they are consenting to and, because of the power structure of the relationship, they do not have the true freedom to say yes or no.[16]

Using Threats and Force

Not all abusers spend time and energy grooming their prey. Several survivors described their experiences as attacks that left them bruised and battle-torn. For Kim (Chapter 2), her stepfather's abuse progressed from grooming to violent sexual and physical attacks. As Kim began to fight, those attacks came with warnings and subtle hints that she or her mother would be hurt if she disclosed what was happening. He eventually wore down her resistance, and for a while she stopped fighting.

WHY SOME CHILDREN ARE AT GREATER RISK

Unless adults are vigilant, all children are at risk for sexual abuse, because an offender needs only an urge, an opportunity, and no resistance. Girls are at greater risk than boys, according to analyses of reported incidents. But researchers stress that boys and men are less likely to disclose that they have been abused, partly because of fears of being stigmatized as homosexual. The next chapter will focus on the issues of Black boys who are abuse survivors.

Experts have identified factors that put some children at higher risk than others. It's clear that abusers thrive in chaotic, stressful situations, as in Carol's home. But Carol's poor relationship with her mother left her even more vulnerable to her father, who had already proven to be physically and verbally violent. Experts emphasize the connection between mothers and daughters; a lack of maternal warmth has been linked with mental health problems, including depression. One study determined that lack of maternal warmth was the strongest predictor of the risk of sexual abuse.[17] Other factors that expose children to greater risk of abuse include:[18]

- **Absence of parents.** Not having parents present exposes children to the whims of caregivers and their associates. Absence could include a parent disabled by substance addiction, emotional, or physical problems. Children in foster care are particularly vulnerable.

- **Poor relationship with parents.** Some studies have shown that molested women were more likely to report having distant, punitive parents.

- **Poor relationship between parents.** Children of parents in conflict may be emotionally needy or deprived, and abusers can seek to fill that void.

- **Stepfather or unmarried male partner in home.** One study determined that a stepfather in the home more than doubles a girl's risk; some experts suggest that stepfathers may not feel a sense of restraint with children whom they have not known and cared for since birth. Another study found that risk increased significantly with a mother's employment outside the home when a stepfather was present.

- **Few friends.** Social isolation from peers and even siblings leaves children vulnerable to abusers who will capitalize on their need for friendship.

- **Lack of information, or negative information, about sex.** When children's natural curiosity about sex and sexuality is not addressed or is punished, they are more vulnerable to victimization because they don't not know what is appropriate and inappropriate sexual behavior.

- **Lack of appropriate physical affection from parents.** Children who do not experience nonsexual touch from adults in their lives are not likely to understand the difference between affectionate touch and sexual touch.

- **Alcohol or drug use in home.** Alcohol and drugs are known to lower inhibitions, enabling a potential offender to act on an emotional or physical need.

- **A history of sexual abuse in the family.** If past abuse has not been addressed, people are less likely to reduce risks or to respond.

These are the more common factors that indicate higher risk. This list is not to suggest that any one factor can lead to sexual abuse, though one study determined that among children with no risk factors in their backgrounds, abuse was virtually absent.[19] Typically, it is a combination of factors that exposes children to potential abusers. In Carol's case, she contended not only with a poor relationship with her mother, but also with a poor relationship between her parents, her father's use of alcohol, a lack of information about sex, few friends, and little nonsexual physical affection from her father.

NO KNOWLEDGE, NO POWER

You simply can't avoid some of life's circumstances, like absence of a mother and the presence of a stepfather. But among the majority of survivors I interviewed, the one risk factor most often cited is lack of information about sex.

In Chapter 1, I briefly explored how our society's reluctance to acknowledge and talk about sex and sexuality leaves a vacuum in our children's minds that is easily filled with images and references from media and their friends. This "information" is usually unrealistic at best and distorted and dangerous at worst. And we so easily pass on to our children our adult hang-ups, often without even realizing it.

Think about it. How did you learn about sex? Did your parents struggle to answer your questions, or berate you or suggest that you were "wild" or "loose" for merely asking? Were they uncomfortable when they tried to answer you? Or did you know from their expressions or body language that you shouldn't even *think* of asking? Which of those responses did you inherit? How do you address your children's sexuality? Is it any wonder that our kids are embarrassed and ignorant about the basic form and function of their bodies when we raise them to refer to certain parts as "coochies," "ta-tas," "wee-wees," and "bum-bums"? We need to help children become comfortable with their bodies—and to set boundaries. If Aunt Sally wants a kiss and your little one resists, don't force the issue. Children pushed to submit to affection may begin to feel that grown-ups' demands are more important than their own physical limits.

THE ART OF LISTENING

Few of us intentionally neglect our kids. Usually what happens is that parents lose focus on their priorities. It's that loss of focus on priority number one—our children's safety and well-being—that keeps us from watching closely and listening intently to what they are telling us. Most survivors described a situation in which their pain and discomfort went undetected as parents or guardians went through the "parenting motions," as one woman describes: from work to home to dinner to bed and back to work again, leaving them feeling as if they were on their own. Few survivors recall actual conversations with their parents; instead they remember orders, directions, and objections. It's almost as if their parents didn't want to know the answers, so they didn't ask the questions.

We must encourage our children to talk to us, and we must cultivate relationships in which they feel free to tell us *anything*. Don't let a fear of shame or ridicule or punishment keep them from confiding in you, says Dorothy Cunningham, the clinical psychologist in New York City. "You can't have closed communication and then expect it to be open if there's sexual misconduct." To cultivate more openness, let your children know that their feelings and opinions are important, Invite them to talk to you, Cunningham said. "Don't just ask, 'How's school?' when you can get a much richer dialogue from 'How's your teacher?' and 'What did you do today?'"

If you tend to get one-word answers, ask your child, "Tell me something you liked about school today," or even "Tell me something you didn't like." One school that I know of has children start each day by indicating their mood on a checklist. They choose from streetlight signals: Green is good, yellow is so-so, and red means watch out! You can adopt a similar system and ask your child her color for the morning or the evening, and then talk about why. Ask about their ever-evolving relationships and friendships, and make sure to give feedback so they know you're listening and responsive.

Also learn to "listen" with your eyes as well as your ears for shifts in mood and behavior. "If you're tuned in, you know when she's upset," Cunningham says. Later on, we'll explore more specifics on what to listen for.

RAISING THINKING CHILDREN

We must help our children develop a strong sense of self and personal boundaries. Their place in this world does not mean that they're destined to fill a preassigned societal role because they're Black, poor, male or female, or young. They need to know that they aren't meant to be "seen and not heard," as our parents may say, because that's how their parents raised them and how they raised us. We need to break with traditions that have stifled us and send new messages to our children. They must know that they are intelligent beings whose words, thoughts, opinions, feelings, and fears matter to us more than anything else.

In order to prevail, our children must be critical thinkers. As soon as they are able to understand, we must encourage them to see themselves not as isolated beings but as part of a society that is constantly shaping their self-image. As Rhea Almeida, the psychologist who heads the Institute for Family Services in Somerset, New Jersey, says, our thinking and behavior are often a product of our culture—movies, music, and television in particular. Almeida's institute uses this cultural context model to teach clients as young as three to recognize how society's messages influence us.

Before they even begin the center's group therapy sessions, clients undergo a cultural context "reeducation," often focusing on popular movies and television programs. In one exercise, Almeida uses characters in the Disney animated film *The Little Mermaid* to explore how we are socialized on issues like race and gender. In the movie, the mermaid Ariel makes a deal with the witch Ursula to trade her tail for legs so she can walk on land with her beloved Eric. Almeida encourages children to discuss the images and messages in the movie. "Of course, the witch is depicted as a big, fat, ugly, dark woman who has the power," Almeida explains. "And Ariel's a pencil-thin, white-skinned girl." She also notes that to be with her man, Ariel must give up her voice, while to be with Ariel, she asks, "What does Eric have to give up?" The answer is nothing.

This approach to communication and self-reflection helps even children see themselves in the context of a White, male-dominated power structure, Almeida says. As parents, we can take a cue from Almeida and use music, movies, and television programs to teach our children to think critically about the world around them. When watching WB's *Men in Black* cartoon, my son remarked, "The brown guy isn't so smart." That opened up a door for a talk on how the people who made the cartoon made the brown character act silly, while his White partner was made to act serious. But, my son agreed, the brown guy chased aliens just as well as his partner.

We then talked about other cartoons, like Bill Cosby's *Little Bill* on Nickelodeon, in which brown characters appear just as "smart" as other characters. Meanwhile, I told my son, he could decide not to watch *Men in Black* if he didn't like how the character was portrayed. I wanted to demystify media stereotypes by explaining that the programs he watches don't just appear but are produced by people and reflect their interests and intentions. I wanted to remind him that he had a choice: He could always turn off the TV, which he often does on his own. In everyday conversations, we empower our children to question and challenge the status quo. Likewise, when we arm them with information about sexuality and sexual abuse, we help them feel more comfortable questioning and challenging those in authority who might make them feel uncomfortable.

Please take note: Teaching children to think critically, to question and challenge, can prompt unsolicited expressions of opinions, intelligence, and confidence. Because of our history and baggage, some Black folk aren't comfortable seeing Black children confidently express themselves and may try to "put them in their place." To some, it's considered showing off, boastful, and even disrespectful. Parents may find themselves supporting and even defending their child's right to be. My young son's ease in conversing with adults caused one relative to snip, "Who does that child think he is?" My answer: "He thinks he is loved. And that his opinions matter." Translation: He's *my* priority number one.

RECOGNIZING SEXUALITY

Part of making sure children are informed and protected from abuse is to acknowledge that they are sexual beings. Note that doing so is not "sex education" but a recognition of sexuality. This may be disturbing for some parents to consider, especially those of us who were brought up to think of sexuality as something dirty or sinful, or who were abused ourselves. Some fear that talking and teaching about sexuality is like giving their children a license to have sex. On the contrary, it is *not* talking about these issues that gives offenders an opportunity to abuse, says the psychologist and certified sex counselor Gwendolyn Goldsby Grant. "You can see why a child who doesn't have any understanding of life would think, 'This happened to me because I was bad,'" she says, when instead, a knowledgeable child might think, "'This happened to me, but it was not supposed to happen, and I'm going to tell somebody who can do something about it.'"

Our children are smarter and more insightful and perceptive than we give them credit for. Many of them at a young age are already forming their own opinions on sexuality by simply watching the adults around them. Surely as a child, you remember being aware of extramarital affairs, unexpected pregnancies and unwanted children, and other family secrets that you weren't supposed to know, but you avoided trouble from the grown-ups by not letting on that you knew. Don't think for a moment that your kids are not playing that same game. Give them the proper information, make sure they understand it, and trust that they will know how to use it.

The key to recognizing a child's sexuality is to put information into context. "We should take everyday opportunities to teach our children about how bodies work," says Grant, a frequent *Essence* magazine contributor. "There is no special time for the birds-and-bees conversation," especially as more than half of all juvenile victims of sexual assault are under age twelve.[20] Grant adds that the "big talk" kind of approach only reinforces a sense of mystery and taboo about sex. "The conversation starts when you're changing his or her diaper. You start by talking anatomy. Touch his toe and call it a toe. Touch her nose and call it a nose. Touch his penis and say 'penis.'"

As they grow older and can understand more, incorporate more complex information. But be mindful of what you say and how you say it. And if you struggle to find a way to say it, get help. "If you feel uncomfortable with the subject, it's OK, because no one laid the groundwork for you," Grant says. "So what you do is you tell a child, 'I'm really uncomfortable with this. My mother never talked to me about it. Let's go to the library, or let's get some books.' Be honest, and you will open doors for the child's thinking for the rest of their life."

Grant credits her mother with informing her practical view on sex education and

Fast Facts

Two good books that explain sexuality are *It's So Amazing! A Book About Eggs, Sperm, Birth, Babies, and Families* (Candlewick Press, 1999), by Robie Harris and Michael Emberley, and for older kids, *The Underground Guide to Teenage Sexuality: An Essential Handbook for Today's Teens and Parents* (Fairview Press, 1997), by Michael J. Basso.

with protecting her. "We're conditioned to think of women in pieces, like parts of a chicken: a thigh, a breast, a leg. But my sex is between my ears. Never has been between my legs, because my mother lifted my consciousness. See, Mama used to say that intercourse is but one little grain of sand on the whole beach of human sexuality. Sex is who you are and how you think, she'd say. It's how you create things—music and art. All that comes out of our creative sexual experiences. And that has nothing to do with sexual intercourse. That's just one little thing that happens."

Grant recounts a time when she was abused as a little girl: "When I was eight, my father used to drive around an old crippled man, who would place a blanket over his legs. I was sitting in the back seat of the car with him one day, when he reached over and pulled my hand under the blanket and onto his erect penis. I snapped around and said loudly, 'My hand doesn't belong on your penis!' with my mouth poked out and my angry green eyes flashing. That man went into an epileptic seizure," she says, laughing at the memory of his surprise. "He never thought a little girl would have a voice. I had a voice."

TALKING ABOUT SEXUAL ABUSE

How do you give children a voice? Simply, directly, and matter of-factly. You can say to your child, "Nobody should touch you there" or "Nobody kisses you on the mouth." And don't be afraid to ask direct questions, such as "Has anyone ever tried to touch you in a way that you did not like, or asked you to touch them in a way that made you uncomfortable?" One woman who was abused by an older relative for years during her childhood says that if her mother had asked her a direct question, her painful secret would have come out.

When Pam Church teaches her powerful Good Touch/Bad Touch® prevention curriculum in classrooms throughout the country, she explains it to kids just like this: "Sexual abuse is when someone tries to force or trick a child into touching that child's private body parts, or into getting the child to touch their private body parts." Then she tells the class to repeat after her.

Just as many of us learned basic rules like "i before c except after c" through repetition, Church encourages children to memorize important rules regarding body safety. Sharing upbeat stories and a multiethnic mix of images that show how children deal with different forms of violence (she addresses bullying, too), Church reinforces to children that they have a right to their own bodies, they have a right to be safe, and they should seek help if they are threatened or harmed. It may seem obvious, but remember that parents rarely take the time to explain these rights, assuming that somehow children know. Church, a child development specialist who has been teaching her curriculum since 1984, sees her role as filling that dangerous void.

"Kids are the only one of the two who will know if a predator enters into their lives," she says. "It's highly unlikely that a parent is going to know, until it's too late." Church says that with her program, "I'm giving kids skills and knowledge, so they have a chance. Because right now, they have no chance at all. There is no way a child could outmanipulate a groomer, who's been practicing and has figured out how to work a child's own good nature against himself. We're giving kids ways to be able to see through the tricks, and to recognize that feeling that says, 'Something feels weird here. I'll talk to somebody I feel safe with about it.'"

I watched Church teach first, third, and fifth graders in a small-town Georgia elementary school for three days, as she trained other Georgia teachers and counselors to take the program back to their own schools. In different lessons appropriate for kindergartners through teenagers, Church describes good touches, like hugs and holding hands, and bad touches, like pinching and kicking. And then she explains, to the little ones, for instance, that there are sexual abuse touches, which "can make us feel sad and yucky on the inside, where our feelings are." She gets children to recognize that they have instincts, and she acknowledges that sexual abuse touches may feel "good or bad on your body," but that touches on private body parts can give children "uh-oh" feelings, warnings that something is not right.

For the fifth graders and above, Church spends extra time focusing on her fourth and fifth Body Safety Rules: "Tell Someone" to make abuse stop, and "It's Never My Fault." These rules get special attention because, she says, their growing independence and sense of autonomy make it more difficult for older children to grasp the concept that someone else can victimize them without their consent.

"By the fourth and the fifth grade, there's a shift," she says. "It's when they naturally take on more ownership and more responsibility for themselves, so the blaming that a perpetrator does is easy, and that's when society begins to blame. The older you are, the harder it is, and the less likely a child is to tell, so we spend a day on why telling is right.

"We role-play, we talk about crime, we do all kinds of stuff to break that denial down."

By the time Church finished her three-day training, it was clear that her young charges were energized with a whole new sense of self: that they were important, that people cared about them, and that they deserved to be heard. You could say that Church is grooming children not to be victims. With her Good Touch/Bad Touch® program, she's teaching them that they have a voice.

I have adapted her curriculum's Body Safety Rules into The Child's Bill of Rights at the end of this chapter (page 148).

SEXUAL VERSUS SEXUALIZED CHILDREN

Not only do we need to recognize that our children are sexual beings, but we also need to acknowledge that their sexuality doesn't start with puberty. Children are curious, and they often explore their bodies. How we respond to that can have lasting impact. My friend tells the story of her five-year-old son, who developed a habit of absentmindedly touching himself in public. "He knows that people have private body parts, that nobody is to touch them but Mom and Dad and the babysitter at bath time," she says, "and that he should tell Mom and Dad about any touch that makes him feel uncomfortable. But teaching him the important social rule of no public touching was a lesson for both of us."

My friend, a sexual abuse survivor, knew her son's habit made her uncomfortable. So before she spoke to him about it, she says, she had to check her own hang-ups first. "I realized that I was afraid that he would be seen as perverse for touching himself, and that I'd be seen as a poor mother for raising a child who would do such a thing." Knowing that five is an age when children are in exploration mode, she says, she never for a moment thought that *he* was the problem; it was merely the perception of others that concerned her. "I wanted him to stop touching himself in public, but I did not want to pass on my issues and alarm him or make him feel uncomfortable. And I didn't want to convey to him that touching his own body was wrong."

So she asked, in a nonconfrontational way: "Sweetie, I notice that you keep touching your penis. Why is that? Does it itch?" His answer threw her for a loop: No, it didn't itch, he said, "but it feels good when I touch the part between my penis and the 'bags' behind it." She says she drew a breath (mostly to give herself time to find the right words and deliver them in the right way) and said calmly, "That's nice if it feels good when you touch it there, but you know, it's not polite to touch yourself on your private parts in front of other people." His response: "Oh, OK." When she recounted the conversation with me she marveled at how matter-of-fact he was about his body. And his habit of touching himself in public has slowly faded away, without any residue of embarrassment.

There's a big difference between being sexual and sexualized. A sexual child is aware of and comfortable within her or his body. Questions may seem naive, observations quaint. But sexualized children will go far beyond simple curiosity and exploration. Their approach to sexuality will be much more sophisticated because *they have been taught* by an abuser.

Sexualized children might reenact behaviors such as tongue-kissing and fondling, and they may seem obsessed with descriptions of sexual perform- ances and acts of sexual gratification. The stepfather serving seven to fifteen years in an Ohio prison for repeatedly abusing his stepdaughter remembers how the child was so conditioned by their sexualized relationship that she would crawl in his lap while watching TV and casually reach for his penis.

IDENTIFYING SEXUALIZED CHILDREN

Teachers and counselors represent a critical line of defense against offend- ers. Because they work so closely with children, they may also see signs or behaviors indicating abuse long before parents notice, or they may see what parents can't or don't know how to deal with.

Carmen Murray, a veteran social worker based at two middle schools in Detroit, has dealt with many of these cases. Often a teacher brings the sex- ual abuse to her attention, and then she, following legal requirements, will report it to Michigan's Department of Child Protective Services. One of Murray's biggest challenges is getting parents to acknowledge and validate the child's experience, and to get help.

She recounts one case, an eleven-year-old boy who seemed obsessed with sex. "He would say things like, 'I made that, I made that' or 'I'm going to get me some,'" she says. "Now, granted, it's middle school, and kids that age do talk about sex, but he seemed to be overboard, inappropriate, and he was the ringleader. It got to the point where the teacher asked if something was wrong because all he talked about was having sex." The obsession, along with poor attendance, led Murray to speak with the boy's mother. And that's when things got tricky.

The mother's first response was to accuse the teacher of "picking on" her son, Murray said. When faced with having to deal with such a horrible and complicated problem, it can seem easier for some parents to go on the defensive. "Sometimes parents deny or get very hostile," she says. "They already feel like they messed up, so to speak. So when somebody brings it to their attention, it makes them feel even worse."

Murray, playing mediator, worked to assure the mother that they were talking out of concern for the boy. After she gained her confidence, the boy's mother shared this: "Don't tell the teacher, but we believe he was fondled by this girl when he was younger." A few weeks later, the family had moved, with a child and his mother clearly in need of help.

In some cases, it is not unusual for a family to disappear after a child discloses abuse, Murray says, because many parents, especially those who are embarrassed or who have something to hide, don't want the authorities in their business. She also recognizes when well-meaning parents don't know what to do, and so they end up doing nothing. "People feel such guilt that they want to do whatever they can to make things better without really dealing with it because it is so painful," she says.

But Murray reminds us of the emotional journey a child has traveled by the time the secret comes out, and how much they need to feel safe and protected. "It's a major breakthrough," she says. "All along they've heard, 'Don't talk, don't tell, don't trust.' So when they do break through, they say to us, 'Don't tell anybody,' and even go over the reasons you can't tell. Because they've been holding on to the secret for so long."

SIGNS OF DISTRESS

While counselors like Murray work closely with teachers to determine when children are in distress, parents can also "listen" with eyes as well as ears for physical signs. Complaints of mouth or throat irritation, pain, redness, itching or burning in the vaginal or anal area, or vaginal discharge should be brought to the immediate attention of a medical professional who specializes in child sexual abuse. Similarly, an onset of a skin or breathing problem, such as a rash or asthma, should receive medical intervention, and special attention if accompanied by any recent mood or behavioral changes.

The challenge is that unless they are obviously sexual in nature, behavioral and attitude changes typically are more difficult to notice. But when a change is abrupt, Murray says, it is especially important to take a closer look. Don't dismiss a surprisingly angry or confrontational child as all of a sudden "acting like she's grown." When children act out, they are trying to get our attention but don't know how to express their distress. In Chapter 2, we touched briefly on how, through their behavior, some children "tell" without verbalizing that they have been abused. Sexually abused children may exhibit these signs, many of which are symptoms of depression:

- Loss of interest or withdrawal from important activities
- Lack of involvement in outside world
- Inappropriate interest in or knowledge of sexual acts
- Hyperactivity
- Rebellion/challenging authority
- Hostility
- Excessive aggression (particularly in boys)
- Regressive behavior, such as thumb-sucking and bed-wetting
- Sleep disorders (nightmares, trouble falling asleep)
- Change in eating patterns, increase or decrease in appetite, nausea, stomach pains
- Passivity
- Self-destruction (cutting, biting)
- Running away, stealing, lying
- Early use of drugs or alcohol

Older children may show these additional signs:

- Early sexual involvement
- Promiscuity
- Delinquency
- Suicide attempts

Instead of acting out, some children "act in," and their changes in behavior can be even more difficult to spot. In Carol's case, her signs of distress were almost invisible.

HIDDEN SIGNS: CAROL'S COPING SKILLS

Carol was in the fifth grade when she learned the definition of incest, in the schoolyard, from a know-it-all classmate sharing her ten years of wisdom.

Carol's reaction: "I was mortified. Probably the most devastating horror of all was the guilt and shame when I found out this behavior between a father and daughter wasn't normal. I remember going home, and I don't think I ate that night. I didn't talk to anybody. I was in total disbelief. How could this have happened? How could I have been taken advantage of in this way?"

It was about that time that her father tried to penetrate her. Carol tried to figure a way out. "I said that it hurt and asked him not to do that," she says. "After that, he returned to heavy fondling or oral sex. Then I said I didn't want to 'play' anymore." He eventually stopped drinking, and stopped the abuse. Then Carol began to blame herself. "The guilt and shame mostly stemmed from being a willing participant," she says. "I never suspected that when he said to just keep it between us that we were doing something wrong. I mean, he was my dad, right?"

With her new knowledge and the feelings of guilt and shame that came with it, Carol felt she had nowhere to turn. She had seen her father berate and beat both her mother and her brother, so she knew that neither of them could rescue her. So she did as they did, and learned ways to mask the mental and emotional pain that came from living in a violent, alcoholic home. The coping strategies that Carol developed helped to see her through childhood, but they would later prove to impair her emotional and social development as an adult. To sexual abuse survivors, these may seem quite familiar:

- **Masking the pain.** "I remained that loud, boisterous kid that the principal was always telling to be more ladylike," Carol says. "Ours is a family of tall secrets. Masking pain with laughter—and we all did it—put up a good façade. No one, not even close family members, knew what was really going on. I clowned in school, church, everywhere. I was so scared of people not liking me if they really knew me or my family."

- **Reaching above and beyond.** "I had to be everyone's best friend," she says, describing a common need to please and be the best to compensate for what's happening at home. "I wanted people to like me, in spite of my secrets. I had to stand out as the good kid, and I had to be active in as much as possible. If I was a good kid, I thought, maybe my family would get better."

- **Avoiding the source of pain.** Carol longed to visit friends and looked to other families as "being a model of real Christian homes," she says. It was rare for her to have her few friends over for anything more than a brief visit. "I hate to think that my dad would have defiled one of my friends for the sake of me having a sleepover." Similarly, a child will find elaborate ways to steer clear of her or his abuser. "The worst thing—or best thing, depending on how you look at it—my parents did was give me a car at sixteen," Carol says. "From then on, I stayed in the streets; mostly over other friends' homes, idolizing their family life, participating in school and church activities and working."

- **Hiding in plain view.** When I interviewed Carol, she proudly shared that she had dropped a dress size. She's been overweight for years, dressing in baggy clothes "in an effort to mask myself as a woman, downplay my femininity," she says. "Mainly to avoid the attention, because if I got the attention, someone might take advantage of me." As she works to heal, she is finding it easier to shed the layers of skin and clothing that she's hidden behind for so long. She's come a long way. These days, she says, "When I do dress up, I know I'm gorgeous."

A LONELY JOURNEY TO HEALING

Carol knows why her mother could not have seen these "hidden signs" as changes in her daughter's behavior. She too was being terrorized, and the fear and isolation of living with a batterer probably obscured her own vision.

Carol used to say that she was amazed that her mother stayed with a man who inflicted so much pain and anguish on her and her children, but now, she says, "I have been counseled that she too may have suffered from childhood sexual abuse and has yet to come to terms with it." But still, she says, empathizing with her mother doesn't lessen the pain or ease her lonely journey.

When she was sixteen and her parents had separated, Carol told her mother about the abuse, hoping that she wouldn't take her father back. Her mother's response: nothing, Carol says. "No ranting and raving, no calls to the police or social services, nothing. And probably the most damaging: no psychological help for me." Her father eventually moved back home. When she was eighteen, Carol told her brother, who had grown distant from the family. His response, "Wow, that's too bad." After that, she vowed not to discuss the abuse with anyone else. "I felt confused, unprotected, stupid, as if no one could understand or help me. I resigned myself to suck it up."

In the mid-1990s, her family went to counseling, primarily to deal with her brother's withdrawal. It was there that Carol learned how everyone had been a part of her abuse. She was stunned. A sharp therapist, who immediately picked up on the family's dysfunction, remarked to her brother, "You're angry," and to Carol, "You're holding a lot of secrets." The therapist suggested that the children ask their parents to explain what they did that hurt their children. Carol reluctantly asked, and to her surprise, her father acknowledged the abuse. "He fessed up," she says, "but he minimized by using the word *molest* and saying that it happened once and that he was drunk." Then the therapist asked her mother and her brother if they were aware of the abuse, and if so, what did they do. They both said yes and that they'd done nothing. Her mother added, "This is an issue between her and her father, and Carol should just get over it." Carol, devastated, has not gone home since.

She felt she had to tell other relatives, particularly an aunt with a six-year-old daughter who spent a lot of time with Carol's parents. Another aunt responded with the disclosure that Carol's father had tried to sexually abuse her, too. An uncle remarked that Carol's family would rather remember fond memories than the "bad stuff." Ultimately, e-mails and calls from relatives trickled to almost none. Carol feels that her family has blamed the messenger. "When I share the secret to get out from under it, I'm somehow labeled a troublemaker or brooder," she says. "Nobody cares about the private hell that I've been through." She's taken a cue from her brother: "Rather than play the charade at family gatherings, I cut everyone off." The feeling of loss is keen especially around the holidays, she says, but it's nothing compared with still feeling violated, "as if they all had been my perpetrators."

Carol moved to San Francisco, where she began to seek spiritual sustenance and healing. She was a lonely, depressed woman who was afraid to trust, who feared the intimacy of friendships with women and relationships with men. At thirty-six, she's never had a boyfriend. She has never made love. She has doubted her professional abilities and has often found herself constantly on alert for any unwanted sexual advances at work.

It was a sermon from Mark 5:25-34, preached by a guest speaker at her church, and an invitation for those who'd been abused to come forward for special prayer and anointing, that helped Carol find her way. "This was the first time I'd seen a church address the issue of sexual abuse publicly," she says. "It was difficult because it was a public statement about something I'd just as soon keep secret." She worried about who would see her but went to the altar anyway, her desire for healing outweighing a fear of being "found out."

The experience made her want to learn more about sexual abuse, and she has built a library of about twenty spiritual and secular books on the subject. She became a lay counselor at church, began to speak at conferences on abuse, and decided to devote her career to her new life's purpose. With her doctorate, she plans to provide therapy to sexual abuse survivors. "My continual healing has come from deciding to be whole and to help others who are stuck in their pain and suffering," she says. "As we continue to talk about and counsel people about such a hideous act as sexual abuse, more people will open their eyes and work to stop it."

HELP YOURSELF

Become a Proactive Parent

It's not enough to teach our children to say no and to tell if they are abused. Adults must take more responsibility to keep them safe. Darkness to Light, an information and education organization in Charleston, South Carolina, distributes a pamphlet, "7 Steps to Protecting Children from Sexual Abuse," which is an excellent guide for not only parents, but also school, church, and community groups. You can request copies of the booklet by contacting Darkness to Light, 247 Meeting Street, Charleston, SC 29401; (843) 965-5444; www.darkness2light.org. These steps are adapted from the guide.[21]

- **Know the facts and the risks.** Be aware of the threat that children face. Make decisions based on the *facts* of sexual abuse rather than a level of trust in others. For example, be aware that disabled children are particularly vulnerable to sexual abuse.

- **Reduce the risks.** Eliminate or reduce one-adult/one-child situations involving your child. If your child is in a one-on-one situation, make unannounced visits, just to check in. Monitor your child's use of the Internet, where pedophiles can interact with children and lure them to meet in person.

- **Talk about it.** Understand why children often keep abuse a secret. Remove barriers that keep them from "telling." Use books or other information if you need help.

- **Stay alert.** Don't expect obvious signs when a child is being sexually abused. Be aware of subtle emotional or behavioral signs of distress.

- **Make a plan.** Know where to go, whom to call, and how to react in the best interest of the child, even if you have no suspicions that the child is being abused. Know that showing anger or disbelief may make the child shut down, change her story, or feel even more guilty. Early planning will help you and the child should abuse ever occur.

- **Act on suspicions.** Be a part of the solution, not the problem. If you have a hunch, act on it; your silence will only contribute to the psychological and emotional turmoil of a child. If you suspect a child is being abused, approach a nonoffending parent or guardian with your concerns and share any information (literature, contact numbers) that you have. If that adult does not act to protect the child, call the police or your local child protective services agency. Do not question the child or approach the suspected abuser yourself.

- **Get involved.** Volunteer for and support organizations that fight child sexual abuse, including prevention programs, rape crisis centers, and child advocacy programs. Ensure that your child's school provides sexual abuse prevention education, which is different from sex education. Also ask the school to provide training for teachers so they can recognize symptoms of sexual abuse. Support legislation that keeps kids safe. Many local sexual assault crisis centers, along with Darkness to Light, can provide information on legislative initiatives. Contact your state lawmakers, and members of Congress, who can be reached online through www.congress.org.

Responding to a Child's Disclosure

Parents should never interpret a child's reluctance to disclose to them as a sign that they are poor parents. Remember that fear of people's reactions and fear of causing family turmoil are two of the main reasons that children don't talk about sexual abuse. For these reasons, children may tell an adult other than a parent. Whether you're a parent or not, if a child does disclose an incident to you, be aware that the appropriate response is critical to their healing. Here are ways you can help:

- **Remain calm.** Don't further injure a child by allowing your anger to show. No matter what you say, she may think your anger is directed toward her.

- **Listen.** Be patient and let her share what she wants in her own way. Don't ask any questions other than "Tell me what happened." Leave the investigating questions to properly trained authorities, who can gather sensitive information in a way that does not inflict further harm or "lead" the child to certain answers.

- **Be supportive.** Tell her how glad you are that she told you, praise her for being brave enough to do so, and assure her that she did the right thing. Don't blame a child for not disclosing any sooner than she did.

- **Believe her.** And show it. Disclosure is often the only way a parent would know a child has been abused. There are rarely telltale signs. A child may see or sense the turmoil the disclosure has caused and "take it back." Recanting is not unusual in these instances. But even so, it is still important to contact the authorities so they can investigate.

- **Comfort.** Say you're very sorry about what happened, and that what happened to the child was wrong. Never suggest that a child encouraged abuse.

- **Reassure.** Tell her that it wasn't her fault.

- **Ensure her safety.** Make sure the offender no longer has access to her. Tell the child that you will do everything you can do to protect her.

- **Take action.** Share information about a case of suspected abuse with others in your family. Put the safety of the child above any family loyalties or allegiances.

- **Report it and get help.** Contact the police, your local department of child protective services (check local listings), or your district attorney's office. Childhelp USA has a National Child Abuse Hotline (800-4-A-CHILD, or 800-422-4453). If reporting abuse does not result in adequate protection for the child, contact Justice for Children (www.jfcadvocacy.org, 713-225-4257). Consult your child's physician, and get a reference for a specialist with expertise in sexual abuse or trauma.

Great Expectations for Every Child

Every child has a right to emotional, mental, and physical safety. The following Bill of Rights is adapted from Good Touch/Bad Touch®, the sexual abuse prevention curriculum developed by Pam Church.[22] Make a copy and use this Bill of Rights to begin or continue a conversation with kids about their basic rights as children. Post the completed document in a prominent place as a reminder. Encourage teachers to use it to start a discussion in the classroom. For more on Good Touch/Bad Touch®, contact PAM Programs, P.O. Box 1960, Cartersville, GA 30120; (800) 245-1527; www.goodtouch-badtouch.com.

The Child's Bill of Rights

I, _____, have a right to know body safety rules. I can determine how I share my body (such as hugs), and whom I share it with (friends, family).

I have a right to trust my own feelings. If I feel like something is wrong, then I am right.

I have a right to question someone's actions, and to ask questions if I am confused.

I have a right to say "No!" and to get away from anyone whose actions make me feel uncomfortable.

I have a right to tell when someone has done something that hurts me or makes me feel uncomfortable. I should tell until someone believes me.

I have a right to be protected from anyone who hurts me or makes me feel uncomfortable. It is never my fault if I am hurt or abused.

I have a right to information that helps keep me safe.

I have a right to put my feeling safe above anybody else's need to keep a secret.

_____   _____
Signed   Date

Adapted from Good Touch/Bad Touch® sexual abuse prevention program.

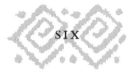

SIX

Helping Boys and Men

I didn't tell my parents till I was thirty-five years old. And even at that point I was
scared. "Oh my God," I thought. "Are they going to think I'm some kind of queer?"

—ROBERT, who was abused as a young boy and as a teenager

ON A LAST-MINUTE DASH FOR POPCORN AT THE MOVIES, I FOUND
myself in line behind a man and his two highly energetic sons, about four
and six. As the father placed his order, the boys took off and circled back to
him in a frenzied game of chicken, running, bumping, tagging, and laughing.
Once the father was loaded to his chin with snacks, he headed toward the theater, and the boys followed, still horsing around, until the little one tripped
and fell, banging his head on the front of the concession stand. The thud of his
fall was loud enough to silence everyone in line. Some people gasped. Some
winced. There was no blood, but you just knew it would leave a bump.

In that moment we've all experienced between the skinned knee and the
tears, the little boy sat up and looked for his father's reaction, as if waiting
for permission to feel. Dad peered down over his pile of popcorn and soda.
"You okay?" he asked hopefully. The boy simply stared up at him without a
word. Finally, the father said, "Shake it off, buddy." Silence. Then the father
asked hopefully, "Can you shake it off?" Slowly the child stood up, rubbing
his sore spot. "You're okay," Dad pronounced, and turned toward the movie,
the older boy fast on his heels. The little one, standing there all alone, knew
he'd get nothing more. He followed silently, still rubbing his head.

I share this story because it shows what our society expects of boys. Shake it off. Tough it out. Suck it up. Be strong. Don't be a baby/sissy/punk. Take it like a man. Boys receive these kinds of messages every day. The overriding message is that they shouldn't feel—unless the feeling is anger or being in control. Many of us impart these views to the boys in our lives, who grow up to become men so grossly out of touch with their feelings (except anger) that they live in an "emotional prison," as one psychologist put it. These men, in turn (and women do their share, too), raise sons who also become inmates in a place where the bars are merely the limits they put on their ability to feel and express emotion. The results are disastrous, individually and for our community as a whole.

MEASURES OF A MAN

American society expects its boys and men to be strong and powerful, brave, problem solvers, defenders and protectors, resourceful, independent, in control. Characteristics such as being kind, considerate, compassionate, empathetic, collaborative, and gentle are not embraced as readily. In fact, in some cases those who display them are considered wimps, henpecked, pussy-whipped, weak.

In some of our neighborhoods, it is dangerous and even life-threatening for Black boys and men to display any of these supposedly feminine qualities. What's left? Boasting or flossing, dissing, and demonstrations of anger and outrage, mostly turned inward toward our own community. For many Black males, especially those who grow up without a responsible father figure to emulate, there can be no more vivid or distorted mirror and teacher of these characteristics than the popular music videos that entertain and, unfortunately, inform young people. Television, along with videos and the Internet, is one of the most important influences on the lives of young people today. And we all know that excessive exposure to violence in entertainment has been linked to increased aggression in children.[1] Spend an afternoon with MTV or BET and you will see one hip-hop video after another celebrating hardened brothers with menacing scowls, bragging about sexual exploits and using violence to make their point.

Of course, much of this posturing is simply a response to the injustices endured by Blacks in America. The hip-hop movement's music, after all, rose up from our streets. In the late '80s it became a popular medium of protest. Through it young artists addressed appalling economic and social conditions—among them high unemployment among Black teens and the Reagan-era assault on youth programs—and reached the masses in a style that was uniquely Black. The content became more violent in the early '90s, mirroring what some artists saw in their homes and communities. These days, however, with rap feuds leading to gunplay and death, it is difficult to determine whether the culture influences the message or vice versa.

The hip-hop posturing that young brothers eagerly mimic also helps them disguise a fear of intimacy with others and themselves. Only a strong sense of self-awareness nurtures intimacy, and intimacy demands "an open, honest vulnerability," as the scholar and author Michael Eric Dyson explains in his essay "Behind the Mask."[2] Dyson writes that many brothers have become so used to using masks to "hide the injuries we've sustained doing battle with society" that "we lose our grip on who we really are." He suggests that home be a refuge, a "no-harm zone," where men can let down their guard and be accepted and understood. But for that to happen, we women, too, need to check our expectations: "Sisters, you often say you want a sensitive man, but when a brother shows his insecurities and fears, you worry that he's going to punk out," Dyson writes. "For a man to get to intimacy, he has to feel safe. It's imperative to communicate that, no matter what he says about his fears and feelings, the relationship can bear it."

"DOES THIS MAKE ME GAY?"

We know that how boys and girls are socialized can profoundly shape their adulthood. Many parents live by the old saying: We raise our sons, but love our daughters. These differences are why I included this chapter devoted specifically to boys who are abused. Studies show no major distinction between males and females in the effects of sexual abuse that they experience: guilt, powerlessness, denial, isolation, depression, sadness, hopelessness, lethargy, and self-destruction, among others. But because of society's expectations, male survivors may struggle particularly with these issues:

- Concerns about sexuality
- Concerns about masculinity
- Isolation
- Feelings of inadequacy and vulnerability

- Recognizing abuse and its effects
- Disclosing the abuse to others
- Finding resources and support

Two of the most common reasons that males don't report abuse are that they don't want to be seen as weak at least and homosexual at worst. Sexual violation has long been a method of emasculation. In ancient times the rape of defeated male enemies was considered a right of conquering soldiers. And a man who was sexually penetrated, even by force, was considered to "lose his manhood" and could no longer be a warrior or ruler.[3]

The question I heard most often from the male survivors I interviewed is "If I was abused by a man, am I gay?" That was followed not too far behind by "Will telling someone about it make everybody *think* that I'm gay?" This is no surprise, given the stigma of homosexuality among African Americans. Often their worst fears were realized when they were not only doubted but questioned or ridiculed. "Did you like it?" one survivor said his own brother asked him after he disclosed his abuse. Can we imagine anyone asking that of a woman who was victimized as a young girl? Society accepts that girls can be victims of sexual violation (though it may blame them for playing a role in their own victimization) because, after all, girls are considered weak and passive.

When boys are victimized, however, the unspoken message is "Why didn't you take care of yourself?" Boys are left to reason that it is best to keep quiet and not expose themselves to further embarrassment or shame.

Fast Facts

- Ninety-three percent of offenders against young males were known to them. Males are more often abused by someone they know who is outside the family.[4]
- Forty percent of boys reporting physical or sexual abuse showed symptoms of depression, compared with 13 percent of boys who had not been abused.[5]
- Abused boys were nearly three times as likely as nonabused boys to show signs of low self-confidence.[6]
- Nearly half (48 percent) of abused boys said they had not talked with anyone about their physical or sexual abuse, compared with 29 percent of abused girls. When asked with whom they shared that they were feeling stressed, overwhelmed, or depressed, boys were more likely than girls to say "no one."[7]
- Abused boys were twice as likely as nonabused boys to smoke or drink frequently or to have used drugs.[8]

And so male survivors of sexual abuse do what they've been taught, and what they see the men around them (if there *are* any men around them) do: They shake it off, they tough it out, and they keep it to themselves, buried under a pile of expectations.

The problem is that the effects of such trauma can't remain buried. Silence cannot hide the fact that sexual abuse is not just a woman's problem: 14 percent of all victims of sexual assault incidents reported to the police are male, and nearly 17 percent of adult men report having been sexually abused in their childhoods.[9]

As estimated with female survivors, males who actually report abuse make up only a fraction of those who are victimized. But the numbers speak volumes: One study shows that 97 percent of offenders who committed violent crimes against children were male, and that violent child-victimizers were substantially more likely than adult-victimizers to have been physically or sexually abused as children.[10] An analysis of studies found that abused males were more likely to sexually abuse others.[11] This is a vicious cycle, enabled by distorted societal messages and sanctioned by silence.

In Black America, severe homophobia—a hatred or fear of gays—perpetuates not only the silence surrounding sexual abuse, but a host of other problems, some of them potentially fatal. Slavery and its legacy have forever warped the lens through which we see Black manhood: If Black men were not able to provide for or protect Black women, the traditional thinking goes, they were therefore less than men. The problem is that this narrow definition, which is shaped by the larger White culture, leaves no room for other forms of Black male identity. Because many of us refuse to acknowledge homosexuality, we will continue to suffer the consequences of men who will not admit that they are gay or bisexual. We've heard the stories of brothers so terrified of being "out" that they hide behind the façade of "my wife and kids" while stepping out with other men on the down-low.[12] This secrecy and denial has not only caused great pain to those who were deceived, but has also contributed significantly to disproportionate numbers of cases of HIV infection and AIDS among Black women.

NOT GAY, BUT PROBABLY CONFUSED

But why would a man think that being sexually abused makes him gay? Let's go back to the messages we send and receive from society: Boys and men are supposed to be strong and self-sufficient. Few can imagine that a male can be forced or tricked into sexual acts. Somehow, the reasoning goes, he must have wanted it or invited it. There must have been something intrinsic in his makeup that made him fair game. Even knowing that he was a child, deceived or overpowered, a male survivor will find it hard to accept that he couldn't have done *something* to fend off an attack. And survivors who are gay must contend with the fact that their introduction to sex with a male was through abuse.

We need to understand that sexual assault has nothing to do with sexual orientation or even an offender's *assumptions* about a victim's sexual orientation. In fact, most sexual abusers are male and consider themselves heterosexual.[13] Sexual abuse is an act of aggression, a violation of power, and a crime of violence in which sex is used as a weapon to hurt, humiliate, or control the victim. Neither attraction, lust, nor passion is the primary motivator for a sexual assault. For many offenders, the choice of a victim is more about access than about sexual orientation, gender, or age.

So to make it clear, the answer to the brothers' question is no—having been sexually abused does not "make you gay." Scientists are still exploring and debating the complex and controversial issue of sexual orientation and how much genetics and environment factor in. What they do know is that, like all early sexual experiences, child sexual abuse is among the many factors that can form one's sexual identity, but it has not been proven to be the sole contributor. But one thing's for sure: while sexual abuse has not been determined to make a survivor homosexual, it certainly can leave him, or her, confused.

In his book *Victims No Longer: Men Recovering from Incest and Other Sexual Abuse,* psychotherapist Mike Lew explores the roots of this confusion: "Survivors tend to worry about sexual feelings of any sort, so that any feeling of attraction toward someone of the same sex can cause great anxiety. It feels like a set-up for abuse. Since all feelings of intimacy are likely to be sexualized, just to *like* another man can feel like a sexual act."[14]

One analysis of studies showed that sexually abused males were up to five times more likely than nonabused males to report sexually related problems.[15] Few men are likely to see the links between sexual dysfunction or confusion and a long-ago victimization.

The situation is just as confusing when a young male's abuser is female (as in 17 percent of instances, according to one survey, compared with 1 percent of cases involving girls).[16] Experts explain that boys underreport abuse by females because they minimize it or dismiss it as a rite of passage. In some instances, there is a tacit acceptance of the violation, often with a wink and nod. Remember society's messages: Girls are supposed to stay virginal and pure, while boys can "get buck wild." In sentencing a forty-three-year-old female teacher to probation for having sex with a thirteen-year-old boy, a New Jersey judge voiced that thinking when he explained why he tossed the three-year prison sentence she was supposed to get under her plea agreement: "I don't really see the harm that was done and certainly society doesn't need to be worried. . . . Maybe it was a way for him, once this happened, to satisfy his sexual needs." Ultimately, an appeals court ordered the woman resentenced, and she got her three years.[17]

Victoria J. Sloan, a clinical psychologist with a private practice in Houston, describes what leads men to rationalize abuse as something they wanted: "A lot of guys I've seen really did not consider themselves victims. Society tells men that if you were a young boy or a budding teen and an adult woman feels you up or has sex with you, then you're lucky. It has to do with those messages that having sex makes you more masculine, more powerful, more of a stud." Once she gets male survivors to move beyond those societal messages and see what actually occurred—"that they had no power and no control over what was happening"—then they are able to recognize that they were abused. Whether victimized by males or females, premature sexual experiences are damaging, with lifelong consequences. Thanks to the courage of men like the author and screenwriter Antwone Fisher, whose book and film shared with the world his powerful story of surviving physical and sexual abuse in Cleveland's foster-care system, more people will come to understand that boys can indeed be victimized by women.

UNTAPPED EMOTIONS

Research has shown that girls display an ability to verbalize feelings before boys. If we raise boys to "shake it off" or penalize them ("Stop crying like a baby!") when they show hurt, or fear, or sadness, they can grow up lacking tools that allow them to connect with and express their feelings. Eli Newberger, a Boston pediatrician and child protection specialist, writes, "When a vocabulary of feelings in young boys is missing in their upbringing, they risk growing up to become men at the mercy of their impulses. They remain unaware of their feelings and inarticulate about them. Until we can apply commonly understood words to things, we can't be fully conscious of them."[18]

Given what little they have left to work with, boys who cannot access their feelings come to understand that they can either be strong or weak, tough or soft, macho or feminine. There's no room for the broad spectrum of emotions and behaviors in between.

The problem is magnified for boys raised without their father or another responsible male figure, as generations of Black boys have been. The writer Ellis Cose explains: "In the worst case those boys end up adopting some supermacho image of masculinity, asserting their manhood by brutalizing other people (particularly the women) in their lives."[19]

When boys are abused, that supermacho image can be a cloak or shield, says Sloan, who emphasizes that unlike her female clients, who seek counseling voluntarily, most of her male clients come because of court action, typically a result of domestic violence charges. "Men work harder to hide abuse than women," Sloan says. "For them, massive energy goes into hiding. That energy causes all sorts of toxic pain, internal discomfort, and agony." Or men get angry, the one emotion that's okay for them to feel, and live "at the mercy of their impulses."

Sloan, who has counseled male survivors as well as abusers mandated for treatment through the criminal justice system, says that to find relief, men often turn inward, medicating or sedating with alcohol or drugs, or they turn outward, to physical and sexual violence. So those music videos that depict brothers inflicting pain are not too far off the mark. Sloan warns parents of abused boys to be especially alert for signs that they are re-creating their abuse with another child. "If you don't resolve the trauma of sexual abuse, you will re-create it over and over, either as the victim or as the abuser," she says. "One of the ways kids compensate for feelings of inferiority or weakness attached to the trauma is that they learn to define power in ways that are associated with the abuser." Where most girls may be terrified and repulsed by abusers and their power, she says, boys more often identify with them and, in their own way of trying to take control of their lives, emulate them by victimizing others.

MEN AT WORK

Who bears the brunt of these behaviors? Family and the community at large. In fact, it is possible to link many of our community's most persistent problems to a history of sexual violence. One analysis found that being abused or neglected as a child increased likelihood of arrest as a juvenile by 59 percent, as an adult by 28 percent, and for a violent crime by 30 percent. Among Blacks, the analysis showed, 40 percent of those neglected or abused were arrested as juveniles, 60 percent as adults, and 34 percent for violent crimes.[20]

Men who beat their wives? Look for a history of sexual abuse. "I often say, 'Show me a man who beats his wife, and I'll show you a man who hates his mother,'" Sloan says. "A lot of this comes out in groups of men who have been charged with domestic violence. They will talk about their mothers who stayed with the man who brutally raped or abused them—and sometimes even witnessed it, but didn't stop it. These men will have a lot of rage toward the women who didn't protect them."

The second wave of feminism forced this nation to recognize the pervasiveness of sexual abuse of girls. Many organizations spotlighted research showing the devastating effects of abuse and created a space for women to come forward, share their experiences, and find resources and help. Since then, many experts have focused solely on the abuse of girls. But as more studies emerge showing the prevalence of sexual abuse of boys, men, too, have begun to find their voices and find help.

The process hasn't been easy, not only because of society's assumptions about masculinity and its homophobia, but also because men tend to be more socially isolated from nurturing relationships than women. But there is hope. Two men share their stories to make it easier for others to do the same. Though their experiences and lifestyles are quite different, it's not difficult to see similarities in the ways that abuse affects our men.

ROBERT'S STORY: TWICE BURNED

Robert, a forty-year-old counselor, lives in Newark, New Jersey, with his second wife and their young daughter. He is the middle child in his family, with an older brother and younger sister. While he was growing up, his dad worked odd hours for the city's sanitation department, and his mom worked for an insurance company. Robert describes his family as "close," but the person he felt he could talk with most was his mother. Dad, he says, led by fear: "I didn't see him much, but we knew that if we messed around, he would definitely give us an ass-kicking."

I ask Robert to describe himself, and he responds with "Warm-hearted, understanding, sensitive." Then he stops and qualifies: "Some people might say, 'Oh, he's too sensitive.'"

Robert's entrepreneurial spirit led him to take up jobs throughout his childhood: After school and summer day camp, you could find him on the streets selling pumpkin seeds, flowers, African beads, newspapers, even Amway.

It was while on his newspaper job that Robert, at fifteen, was fondled by a man who managed the paper route. Though it was not the first time Robert had been abused, it was the first time he kept quiet. With the first experience, Robert was only five, but he had no problem telling his mom about how his dad's best friend "put me on his lap and started humping me." His mother chased that man out of the house with a knife, then promptly told his father, and the "friend" was banished from the family. But why couldn't he tell about the second molestation? At first, Robert says he doesn't know. Perhaps with age came a greater sense of autonomy, as Pam Church suggests in Chapter 5, and Robert felt more responsible for what happened to him. But perhaps because as a male, he was trying to live up to all of those expectations that we have of boys and men. Whatever the reason, Robert managed to block that secret out—until a few years ago. All the while, it seared him deeply. What he remembers about that time is this:

"It happened at least twice. It might have been more. But there were two times that I know. I would go to his apartment to pick up the papers. Ride my bike or push a shopping cart. My parents didn't know him. He used to let me drive his car. He kept promising me I could drive his car. I would do this trick. I would put stacks of coins on the back of my forearm and I would catch them, like thirty at a time. He said, 'Oh, that's great. You're so quick. I'll teach you how to play some basketball or boxing or something. Come by the apartment.' So I went by the apartment.

"He had a gun. It wasn't a real gun, but one of them starter pistols. And he had a tape recorder. And he would fondle my penis. There was no penetration, but he would touch my penis. And he would show me the gun and the recorder. He would talk as he held the gun. He would say stuff and I would answer. I can't remember exactly what we said, but I know he was trying to make it seem as if I was a willing participant. Of course you couldn't see the gun on tape.

"Another time he took me to the office and put me on a table. It was dark. He told me, 'If you get an erection, I'll give you a hundred dollars.' I said, 'Bet. I need a hundred dollars.' I didn't get an erection, though. I just was turned off by it. Because as he was touching my penis, I was like, 'What the hell is happening?' I didn't like that feeling. I didn't know what to make of it. I didn't know if it was normal. I knew I didn't like it. I didn't like being tricked.

"I blocked it out of my mind for twenty years—didn't speak about it until three years ago. The way I remembered it, I was bike riding and talking with my colleague about work. And I got this flashback. And I said, 'Damn. Do you know what happened to me twenty years ago?' Then I had a good cry. He was the second person I told, after my first wife. I just didn't want to tell nobody about that. I didn't tell my parents till I was thirty-five. And even at that point, I was scared. 'Oh my God, are they going to think I'm some sort of queer? Or did I like it? Or what? Are people going to think I'm weird?'"

When Robert told his first wife, it was a painful time for both of them. "She was telling me she was abused," he says. "She was going through so many emotions, and I was like, 'I'm in that boat myself.' I said, 'I'm going to tell you something real quick, and I don't want to talk about it.' I didn't know how to deal with a situation like that.

"That's what helped break up our marriage, her abuse, my abuse, a whole history of abuse. Both of us asking for comfort, but neither able to give it."

Robert now realizes that he didn't know how to help because he was confronted with his own painful past. "I wasn't supportive at all. I just didn't know how to deal with any of it. It was all new to me. What bothered me most of all was opening up, communicating. When we were girlfriend/boyfriend for three years, everything was pretty cool. As soon as we got married, everything went downhill. I assumed she expected more out of me. But I wasn't opening up, really. I was just there."

With his second wife, it was easier to open up. "I've known my wife since she was eight and I was twelve," he says. "She was always my friend—we just happened to hook back up later on in life. I forgot how it happened. I think we were just talking about my job—dealing with child abuse prevention. And I just came out and told her. I said, 'I'm going to tell you something,' and she told me that at one point she was fondled by an older gentleman at her job when she was working at Burger King. She gave me a hug. Tried to comfort me. Told me it wasn't my fault. She said all the right things. She didn't freak out. And she's never thrown it back in my face. She has definitely been by my side."

It was his need for openness and to protect children that led Robert to tell his family.

"I didn't feel a need for it to be a secret anymore," he says. "And I wanted them to be aware of what can happen. People you think you trust, those are the ones who are actually doing it." Looking back, he is sure he wasn't that newspaper man's only victim. "He used to be with other little kids all the time. My brother has a six-year-old son and a three-year-old daughter, and I want him to be aware of what's happening. It happens to a lot of people. I wanted him to know that it happened to me."

When Robert told his parents, he says, their first reaction was anger that he had not told them sooner. His sister was supportive, but his brother— well, telling his brother hurt. "I was hesitant to tell him," Robert says, "he's such a jokester. And of course the first thing he said was, 'Did you like it?' I wanted to punch him in the face. Then he asked if I know where the guy lives. Of course I don't remember where the guy lives. He's probably dead by now, anyway."

As a counselor working with sex offenders, Robert is now a healer. It's not odd that he ended up in this calling, but there was a time when his life could have gone either way. When he was younger, he drifted, he digressed, he destructed. He sees that many of his problems were linked to the abuse and the silence and how he chose to cope—or not cope—with it. "I had problems expressing myself," he says. "I would always hold things in, keep it to myself. I'd think I could medicate it myself. And of course it took years to find out you can't medicate yourself. I don't think I thought of it as bad as it actually is. But it was. Depression. My grades in school."

At some point, he let go of his dreams of being an entrepreneur. He didn't want to go to school, but he knew he wanted to make money. "I tried to sell drugs, I stole cars, I tried armed robbery," he remembers. "Breaking and entering. Hanging with the bad crowd. Just fucking up. It wasn't that I was trying to kill myself, but I was probably reaching out, calling out for help. I didn't know how to call out for help, and I was just doing everything. I never got caught for doing those things, but I was calling for help in the wrong way."

An after-school boys' program proved to be a lifeline. And after several odd jobs, a mentor convinced him to go on to community college. There, Robert gravitated toward counseling. And through the work of helping, and even calling out those who don't own up to their actions, he's found healing and hope.

"Being a victim of sexual abuse affects the work I do," Robert says. "I try to make sure that I'm doing a correct job, make sure that these individuals aren't just coming here thinking that they can pay and get their way out of jail. I'm making sure that they're speaking about the emotions and the feelings that led to the actions, so it won't happen again. I'm always challenging their thoughts, because they always feel that they're the victim, that 'if he or she wasn't dressed in an inappropriate way or hadn't touched me in a certain way, then I wouldn't have done that.' I say, 'Don't hand me that stuff.'"

Nobody gets over. With tough talk and tactics, he makes his point again and again: "I go online and get articles about men being raped in prison. And I read those to my clients. And let them know, 'Don't think because you're 225 pounds and six foot two it can't happen.' They say that if a person is being abused, they want to be abused because they like it, because it's sex. They've got this misconception. Then I go into role-playing, and I'll ask one of the big guys up in group, 'Stand up for a second.' The guy stands up. I say, 'These two guys right here, they're my bodyguards. And I want to stick my dick in your ass. Would you like that?' The answer is no. So I'm always stressing to them that victims don't like what's happening to them. I'm always telling them, just because someone didn't cry rape immediately doesn't mean rape didn't happen, and it doesn't mean they liked it."

In many ways, Robert sees his work as his therapy. He has shared with some of his counseling groups that he is a survivor of sexual abuse. "I know I ain't got to prove nothin' to nobody. But every once in a while I get those strange looks, as if, 'How could you let something like that happen to you?'"

Counseling takes its toll. "When I was running a therapy group at work, the guys were talking about their victims," he says. "Some of their victims were children. And I was getting more flashbacks. I thought, 'Damn, should I hate these guys? Or should I help them?'"

It is a never-ending battle, because sexual abusers can never be cured of their compulsion, only taught to control it or medicated into managing it. "When I go home after groups, when my wife is sleeping," Robert says, reflecting on his role as a survivor and a healer, "I just go for a walk. I clear my head. I meditate. Because hearing about deviant sexual behavior for hours drives me crazy. I try to have hobbies, try to get my mind clear. And I definitely keep God in my life. I listen to sermons on cassette tapes—I have church up in the car. I pop in a cassette and clear my head. Because all this deviancy is sickening."

But even with his knowledge and expertise, even with the lessons he uses each day to try to teach abusers how not to victimize, and even with trying to find healing in the work that he is doing, Robert still struggles to keep those expectations in check. Even today he still questions, doubts, and wonders what if.

"Sometimes I think, how could I have been so stupid? Why didn't I have my guard up? Did I really want this to happen to me? Then I try not to think about it.

"It was hard for me to talk about it. Actually, the first ten times were hard. I think now it's maybe time number sixty, sixty-five. It's getting a little easier. Why didn't I tell? That gun did scare me. But I also didn't want anybody to think that I brought this onto myself. That I was a homosexual." He pauses. "Man, if I was penetrated, that would have really freaked me out. I was always sure about my sexuality. I never questioned it. I'm not homophobic. But after that, when guys would try to come on to me, I'd get very defensive. I don't play that. And I know I wouldn't let that happen to me again."

WILLIAM'S STORY: A BROTHER'S BROKEN TRUST

When I sit down to interview William, a fifty-five-year-old computer technician from the midwest, it doesn't take long to see how deeply he has been wounded—not only by his brother's sexual abuse but also by his parents' emotional abuse and neglect, much of which seemed to be fueled by their own self-hatred. Growing up as the second oldest in a family of three boys and a baby girl, he was an all-A student in a household where A's had no value. William longed for love and affection and for acknowledgment that he mattered. He found them, but at great cost.

William's father worked for a city government, and his mother, a homemaker, was involved with the PTA. From the outside, all seemed well. "My parents weren't exactly socially conscious, but they were community-conscious," he says. "They worried about what people thought. Everybody knew us in the neighborhood, and my dad practically ran his department at work. All the White guys and Black guys were afraid of him."

Inside William's home were fear and dread. "I don't ever remember any good times," he says. "There was always trauma behind everything. My father was the commander. It was speak when spoken to. And if you had anything to say, it was wrong. If I got up and walked through the kitchen and I didn't say good morning, I got slapped down. I was petrified of him. Physically, verbally, everything. I walked on pins and needles all the time. Because any time I said something wrong, I got beat or yelled at."

He never received affection from his parents. "I never got any touching from my mother or father. No embraces, no hugs, nothing. You hug my mother and she would just knock you off." Though his mother wasn't much comfort, he felt safer with her.

William remembers experiencing a form of emotional abuse that has its roots in the self-defeating messages that our ancestors received during slavery. "A nigger ain't shit," his parents would remind him every so often, especially when he seemed to be succeeding beyond their grasp. "Even though you would venture off and do good, you're still a nigger, whether you're brilliant or not. In my house it was not okay to be smart. My dad used to beat me when I brought home all A's. He'd say, 'You think you so smart. Well, I'll show you that you're not too smart. Get out there and clean up. You cheated. You lied. You making them teachers give you all A's, because you're a liar.' It made me feel bad about myself. But I had God in my life, and I said, 'God, I want to make all A's. If I get my ass whipped, I get my ass whipped.' I guess if you want to accept that a nigger ain't shit, then hey, you go ahead and accept it. And you won't be. I think a lot of Black people accept that. I never thought it was true."

He doesn't remember how his brothers and sister fared in this climate of fear, but he knew that he was his father's least favorite. Perhaps because his skin was darker, like his mother's, he thought. Or perhaps because he defied their predictions that he wouldn't be "nothing other than a nigger." Or perhaps because, unlike other little boys he knew, he would rather talk than fight. "I didn't want to beat up on anybody. I always thought that there had to be another solution besides kick somebody's butt." As early as three or four years old, William says, his father called him a girl. "He'd introduce me as, 'This is my little girl William.' Once I finally asked him, 'Why do you call me a girl? I know the difference between a girl and a boy.' He said, 'Because I want to.' I was thirty-eight years old when my daddy first called me a boy.

"I got labeled early," he says. "I guess because I never could hold back my emotion. But every Black man is emotional. And they hold it back, so it turns into something else. They counter it by being mean. And then what does that do? That throws you off from being who you are. I always felt like I don't want to hide."

When he was twelve, his mother suggested that he might be gay. "She told me, 'The more you hide it, the more it's going to show,'" he said. "Well, I was so upset about it. I was about twelve years old, and I said, 'Oh my God. What am I going to do now? I'm already messed up as it is. My dad is messing over me. I'm an A student and nobody likes A students. And now I'm homosexual!'"

The one person he knew he could count on was his older brother, Michael. "I really needed somebody," he says. "I trusted him. I could talk to him. He was my savior."

Michael also became his abuser. William was twelve when his brother, then sixteen, first approached him. The abuse continued for three years. "We would get into bed and be under the covers and fondle and touch," he says. "I don't say it was anal or penetrative. But it was the whole act of touching, and it's your brother. I don't know how that started. All I know is it started, and he continued until he went off to college.

"I never thought it was sexual. To me, it was like we were bonding. It was like divided you fall. My brother's the only person I've got. So to me this was a way of showing love."

The boys' younger brother, who was younger than William by five years, also shared the bedroom. It was clear that he had a sense of what his brothers had been doing. After Michael left for college, William says, the youngest climbed into bed with him. "I told him, 'We don't do that. The buck stops here.' And so we never had any sex. I wasn't about to pass that on. How I knew to do that I don't know."

When Michael sent a letter from college with a picture of his girlfriend, William was shocked and hurt. "That said he was not in love with me," he says. "And all of a sudden, I realized I was out here all by myself.

"Oh, I was hurt, and didn't know who to talk to about it, or where to talk about it. Who could you talk to? You can't talk to your preacher, you can't talk to your teacher. Who can you tell that you've been having sex with your brother for three years? Who'll believe you?"

About that time, alcohol entered his life. "I was sixteen," William says. "It was at a dance in our community where everybody got dressed up. A guy offered me a rum and Coke. I became instantly in love. I did a little drinking while I was still at home, but it would be all over my breath. And my younger brother would say, 'Go upstairs! Go upstairs, because they'll smell it.'"

William's A's eventually landed him a four-year scholarship to a university, where he was one of the first Blacks on campus. There he managed his course work, joined the band, protested at sit-ins, and forged relationships, all without a word of acknowledgment from his parents. "No money for books or anything. No support at all. I don't know—maybe they felt I was outdoing them. I always felt like my parents were in competition with me or something. So I could never feel proud of it, because when you get home, you would get beat about it."

On campus, he drank everything he could. "I don't know if I drank originally to forget, but it helped." Eventually alcohol led to weed and acid in the '70s. In the next decade, there was cocaine, and then crack. For years after college, his life consisted of presenting a respectable front to the outside world while living on the edge. He held jobs, joined a band, and kept up a busy social schedule, but it was the alcohol, and later the drugs, that kept him going and clouded his judgment on relationships. He lost touch with his family— fell out with his younger brother and sister—and his mother died. That left him more alone than ever before.

He struggled with his sexuality. "I had girlfriends, because back in college, you had to have a woman. And I've had some decent relationships with women. But—maybe I thought it was a childhood thing, that if I went to bed with as many women as possible, that that would kill it. And I think a lot of Black men think this way. And I think that's why a lot of Black men have five or six women, trying to kill it. And I tried. Tall women, short women, fat women, White women, Black women. I tried it all. And then it just hit me that, you know, 'You're gay, Will.' Now I have no problem with it. It's like anything else. I can't stop being Black, and I can't stop being gay. I don't advertise it, but I don't hide it, either.

"I want a relationship, and I haven't given up the idea of having a partner, but I'm still afraid of men. During the drinking it was a lot of sexual stuff. They were hustlers. And I guess I'm afraid of the hustlers. You know, guys who know you're gay, come on to you, and you have to pay them to have sex. That was much of my sex life, where I was ripped off, and the honesty wasn't there. I guess it's not that I'm afraid; it's just that I don't want to be messed up. Most men, they can't get honest. Because if you get honest, then you're weak. If you show your emotions, you're weak. And that's if you're gay or straight."

In September 1991, a close brush with death showed William that he wasn't really living. While playing a set with his band, one guy had a heart attack. William, who knew CPR, gave him mouth-to-mouth resuscitation. "I saved his life," he says. "But when I came out of that, I could only think, 'My God, when are you going to save your own life? When are you going to do something for you, Will?' I had learned never to do anything for me. I mean, if I do something for me, then I'm ego-tripping. That's what I was told.

"I realized I was sick and tired of getting high. And I kept telling myself, 'Will, you're letting this drink, you're letting this weed, you're letting this crack just ruin you. When are you going to do something about it?'"

Through his union at work, he found a counselor who recommended therapy.

"My therapist was the first person I told about the abuse. Well, I did tell some people in college, but nobody would believe that a man could be abused. And I had begun to feel like, 'OK, Will, maybe it didn't happen. Maybe you're just making this all up.' You know, your mind be trying to help you. Denial is very positive at the right time. Then some people would say, 'Get over it. It happened a long time ago.' I think we all do that. 'Get over it,' instead of dealing with it, going back to the person, saying, 'Hey, you did this. I don't like this.'"

Therapy helped him understand and articulate his pain. He found Mike Lew's book for male survivors of sexual abuse, *Victims No Longer,* and took the exercises to heart. "I did everything that book said," he says. "He said scream, I was in my house, turned up the music, 'Aaaaaaaahhhhh!' He said to write. And so I wrote. And I think that was the hardest part. Because I didn't accuse, I wrote what happened."

He sent letters to his father and brothers. An outpouring of years of sadness and anger, each ended up about nine pages.

In his letter to his brother Michael, William says, "I told him that that was my first sex. I told him, 'You were the older brother. You could have stopped it. But you were the one who kept it going.' And I said, 'You are the abuser. I keep thinking that I maybe pushed myself on you or forced myself on you. But the bottom line is, our relationship ended the day we started having sex. And I kept on hoping and praying and trying to be a brother. We used to talk about things. But once we started having sex, there was no more conversation.'" No one ever responded to William's letters.

William has been sober since 1992. He ended therapy in late 2001. He is proud of how far he has come and wants to share the lessons that he has learned: "I would say to any man who has been sexually abused as a child to find somebody that you can talk to. Find somebody you trust.

"And find it in your heart to forgive yourself. When my daddy was beating me, I used to say, 'God, I forgive him.' As a child, they told me that whatever you hate, you become. So I said, 'Oh God, I don't want to become my daddy, so I'm not going to hate him. And I don't hate my mama and I don't hate my brother.' But I hated me. For being angry at me, and not being angry at the people I should have been angry with. I've forgiven myself for even thinking how bad I must have been.

"When my therapist said that my mother and father lied to me, I cried. That I'm no good, that I'm worthless. That I don't deserve the good things in life. That I'm a girl, I'm a sissy, I'm a punk. It's hard to accept that your parents lied to you. It just hurt. Because I'd been making them the greatest human beings in the world. But then, when I let go of that, then I started thinking I'm the greatest person. And it's wonderful to work at finding out who you really are. And then accepting it. And then growing upon that.

"I'm fifty-five and I think my life has just begun. Because I don't take shit off of nobody no more."

COMMON GROUND

Though Robert's and William's experiences differ significantly, they have much in common:

- A sense of isolation
- Poor relationship with and fear of father
- Self-blame
- Use of alcohol or drugs to mask pain
- Resorting to destructive behavior as a response to violation
- Trouble developing and maintaining intimate relationships
- Struggles with sexuality
- Struggles with issues of trust

These issues can be addressed through counseling. Parents who might dismiss the need for boys to get help (don't think for a moment that they can "shake it off") are doing them a great disservice. Counseling is critical to help them recognize that they were taken advantage of, that they were not at fault, and that it is okay to have feelings about their experience and to talk about them. And early intervention can break the vicious cycle of abuse and silence. Many pedophiles often begin in adolescence; 23 percent of offenders in assaults reported to law enforcement were under the age of eigh-teen.[21] Through counseling, survivors can learn that they don't have to identify with and adopt the power that was exploited over them. And they can declare, as William did when his little brother climbed into bed with him, "The buck stops here."

In the next chapter I will explore what for many survivors is a significant step in the healing process: challenging abusers.

HELP YOURSELF

Give Encouragement and Support

Male survivors should recognize that in order to deal with the effects of sexual abuse, they must communicate their feelings. For many men, that can be like exercising new muscles. It can be frightening, too, because sharing such experiences can leave them feeling vulnerable and exposed to ridicule or judgment. It may be useful to review the "Help Yourself" exercises in Chapter 5 ("Protecting and Saving Our Children") and explore those in Chapter 4 ("'Getting It Out' and Healing"), but below is additional help for male survivors in particular.[22]

For Parents / Caregivers

If a child reports sexual abuse, immediately contact the police or your local child protective services agency, and make sure he is safe from the abuser. Parents should request a counselor who has experience treating male survivors. Counseling is critical because it helps boys regain a sense of control over their lives. To provide the best support, parents and caregivers need to check their own attitudes about masculinity and sexuality, and monitor the messages they send to their sons. They need to let boys know:

- "You did the right thing to tell."
- "Being strong is being able to say, 'This happened to me.'"
- "Being strong is about getting help."
- "Talking about it helps you get better."
- "It's okay to talk about your feelings."
- "You will be kept safe from the abuser."
- "Being abused doesn't make you gay."
- "Abuse doesn't happen because you're gay."
- "You didn't deserve what happened to you."
- "You're not weird."
- "Abuse is never, ever your fault."

Keep in mind that authorities are not always sensitive to male sexual assault survivors. It may be useful to have a male friend or advocate with you to provide support and assistance when dealing with officials.

For Male Survivors

For men, who are raised to be protectors in our society, one of the most powerful motivators for disclosing sexual abuse is that doing so can help them play an active role in stopping it. As more male survivors acknowledge that sexual abuse is not just a women's problem, and that they are not alone, more of them can speak up and help end the cycle.

Men should take these steps to deal with sexual abuse:

- Seek professional counseling (for the reluctant, a first step could be to call a local or national hotline and inquire anonymously). Ask for someone with experience in treating male survivors. These are the benefits of counseling for adult male survivors:
    - Provides intervention and support
    - Addresses problems that stem from gender and sexual identification
    - Helps understand abuse in context of power, not sex
    - Explores impact of childhood experience, upbringing, and vulnerability
    - Addresses relationship problems
    - Explores issues of sexuality
- Join or organize a support group (do this with the guidance of a mental health or spiritual adviser). Many professionals strongly advocate undergoing one-on-one counseling before or at the same time as group counseling, because the group dialogue may raise issues that cannot be addressed within the group setting or a limited time frame. Here are the benefits of a support group:
    - Helps overcome isolation
    - Helps lessen the impact of the stigma associated with the abuse of males
    - Provides an empathetic, nonjudgmental forum for men to share feelings
    - Helps counteract society's expectations and messages
    - Offers mutual encouragement and understanding

Women Helping Men

Women need to encourage the men in their lives to seek counseling to resolve issues behind destructive behaviors. Women also need to do their part to create a safe space, where, as the writer Michael Eric Dyson says, "No matter what he says about his fears and feelings, the relationship can bear it." If you suspect that a man in your life is a survivor of sexual abuse, raise the issue of abuse in general (use recent news articles or TV broadcasts as a jumping-off point) to provide an opportunity for him to share. If he discloses abuse, here is how to respond:

- Listen.
- Don't offer judgment or commentary.
- Express your concern that he had such an experience.
- Suggest professional help.
- Let him know that you're there if he wants to talk some more.
- Be patient; let him find his way in his own time and on his own terms.
- Maintain his confidence.

Men Helping Men

Brothers desperately need to create their own safe havens, where they can let down their guard and communicate with one another without fear of ridicule or embarrassment. Organized forums such as church groups and fraternal organizations provide excellent fellowship opportunities to deal with issues from intimate relationships to workplace drama. Men who have not been abused must become advocates for survivors by finding ways to support them. Here are a few:

- Be especially sensitive to issues that male survivors struggle with (concerns about sexuality, masculinity; feelings of vulnerability; fear of being considered gay).
- Acknowledge the courage and strength it has taken for them to disclose that they were abused and to seek help.
- Listen.
- Don't offer commentary or judgment. Don't question their actions or thinking.
- Become an activist or a healer. Join a local abuse awareness organization and learn of ways to help survivors in your community.

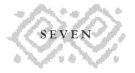

SEVEN

Challenging Abusers

He apologized and I don't hate him. But when he gets out,
I don't want to see him.

—KARLA, nineteen, whose stepfather, Charles, is serving seven to
fifteen years in prison for sexually abusing her

AFTER READING MY ARTICLE IN *ESSENCE* MAGAZINE ABOUT HOW
survivors of sexual abuse can heal by speaking out about their past,
Brenda, a mother of four in northern Ohio, wrote me: "In 1992 the carpet
was pulled out from under me and my children" when her eldest daughter
told her that her husband had been sexually abusing her youngest daughter
for almost four years. "I immediately packed up and moved me and the kids
in with my mother. Then I called a friend who was an attorney." Brenda's
husband, Charles, is now in his eighth year of a seven-to-fifteen-year sentence at a medium-security state prison for the repeated molestation of
Brenda's daughter and his stepdaughter, Karla. Karla was ten when the
secret came out.

Their story is highly unusual. Most situations like theirs never see the
light of day. Experts say that of the incidents of child sexual abuse that are
reported, only a fraction of the cases are referred to the police and to criminal prosecution, and less than 10 percent of the prosecuted cases lead to a
conviction.[1]

Because of fear, embarrassment, and some of the many other reasons
I have explored in earlier chapters, such as not wanting to send another

Black man into the criminal justice system, well-meaning adults might feel that a warning will be enough to keep an abuser in check. They may feel that the threat of public embarrassment will force an abuser to keep his behavior under control. They may decide that they will be on guard, watching for telltale signs to keep abuse from happening again.

But as we've heard from survivor after survivor, these tactics do not work, and they leave children exposed and vulnerable. For many abusers, the boundaries, rules, and laws that society has set up to keep us from infringing on others' rights are not enough to limit their behavior. Many of them even understand that touching or having sex with children is illegal and morally wrong, but understanding is not enough to keep them from acting out. Their sexual compulsions simply override any sense of guilt or embarrassment, reasoning or logic.

Bill Ford, a clinical social worker who is cofounder of Mustardseed, a counseling service for sexual abusers in Brooklyn, explains the mind of a child sexual abuser: "Many of them will clearly let you know, 'Look, I know it's wrong to have sex with my stepdaughter,'" he says. "They will say, 'I understand she's a child. But when my wife isn't giving me sex, when I'm not going out and getting sex from anyone else, when she's available and she's sitting right on my lap, the feeling against my penis is just so arousing that—it just happens.'"

In this chapter, we will focus on abusers to help understand what leads them to victimize and how it can be stopped. It may be disturbing and even painful for you to hear from sexual offenders. But I offer their experiences, as well as the expertise of those working with them, to give us insight into the complex nature of the paraphilias or sexual deviations that often lead to sexually abusive behavior, and to help us protect our children.

WHAT MAKES ABUSERS TICK

In Chapter 5 ("Protecting and Saving Our Children"), I explained some of the more common tactics of child sexual abusers and the four preconditions that enable abuse to occur: (1) There must be a potential offender who seeks a child out for sexual relations. (2) The potential offender must overcome internal inhibitions against acting on this desire. (3) The potential offender must overcome external obstacles or prohibitions against abusing. (4) The potential offender must overcome or undermine resistance by the child.[2]

The first two of these preconditions point to the dysfunctional behaviors of abusers and their relentless drive to engage in sexual activity with children: seeking children out for sexual relations and overcoming internal inhibitions against acting on this desire. Most untreated sexual abusers are unable to resist the impulse to approach and attack. Their drive is fueled by a need to wield power over their prey, and it is difficult to control without professional help.[3] Think about it: Who willingly gives up power? This explains why few people with a sexual compulsion are motivated to seek help on their own, especially if they are able to continue their abuse unchecked.

While sexual abusers differ in many ways (their levels of impulsiveness and persistence, for instance), they do have characteristics in common. Here are some fundamentals about many of them:

- Sexual behavior disorders are chronic, meaning that they are long-lasting and the compulsions can recur frequently.

- Many pedophiles (specifically, those with fantasies, urges, or behaviors involving sexual activity with children thirteen or younger) often start in adolescence; 23 percent of offenders in assaults reported to law enforcement were under the age of eighteen.[4]

- The urge to abuse is complicated or exacerbated by drug and alcohol abuse, depression, stress, and an inability to engage socially with peers.

- Many sexual predators lack the ability to feel empathy for their victims.

- Like substance abusers, few sexual abusers recognize that they have a problem, and few willingly seek help.

- Few child sexual abusers tend to be violent, which makes them difficult to catch and thwart.

- Most operate in silence and isolation, the same tools they use in targeting and controlling their prey.

- Many are manipulative and conniving; like con artists, they lie convincingly and with ease.

These fundamentals make it clear why sexual offenders need to be assessed and managed by professionals who are familiar with their particular perversions and tactics. Nobody knows how many child sexual abusers there are, but as the American Psychiatric Association says, the large child pornography market suggests that the number of people at large in the community with sexual perversions that could lead to child sexual abuse is likely to be higher than studies show.[5] One thing that is for sure: The number of those in state prisons for sexual abuse has increased significantly in recent years.[6]

SUPERVISION AND TREATMENT

Because sexual abusers generally don't turn themselves in, the most effective way that society has found to deal with them is through the criminal justice system, that is, once they have been caught. However, the management of offenders lacks critical funding and staffing in spite of an increase in the number of those convicted of sex offenses. And programs have only recently begun to reflect input from victims' rights advocates.[7] But the system can certainly be expanded and shaped by public pressure. Community notification programs are but one example of lawmakers' response to the public's demands, in this case, to know that a convicted sexual abuser has moved into the neighborhood. You too can press your local representatives to develop strategies to address this complicated problem in your community.

At least one organization is taking a new approach to prevention. Stop It Now, in Haydenville, Massachusetts, challenges abusers themselves to come forward and get help. In a departure from survivor-focused advocacy of most prevention efforts, Stop It Now offers forums not only for survivors but for abusers to talk about their actions and to educate the public. It has run public awareness campaigns and provides a toll-free phone number for potential abusers to call before they act. Stop It Now's approach marks a huge shift in the field of sex abuse prevention, experts say.[8] The group's contact information is listed in Resources.

Currently, the primary emphasis is on abusers once they're in the system. And short of locking all sexual deviants up for the rest of their lives (an expensive and unrealistic solution), experts in the burgeoning profession of sex offender management have a two-pronged approach to prevent them from reoffending: supervision and treatment.

Supervision can be incarceration or, for those on probation or parole, regular contact with a corrections officer. Typically these officers are trained specifically to work with sexual abusers. In some overburdened (big cities) and rural areas, "contact" could mean the offender corresponds with the

Fast Facts

- Two-thirds of state prison inmates convicted of sexual assault had committed their crime against a child.[9]
- Child sex offenders tend to victimize more often than other sexual offenders. Seventy percent of child sex offenders had between one and nine victims; 23 percent had between ten and forty victims.[10]
- Experts say that adolescents, who commit 23 percent of sex offenses, are more responsive to treatment than adults.[11]
- In one study, the number of prisoners sentenced for sexual assaults other than rape increased by an annual average of nearly 15 percent—faster than any other category of violent crime.[12]

officer by mail. Treatment consists of psychological counseling, either alone or with medication that diminishes sexual urges and impulses, or in more severe cases, shock therapy. Treatment often includes help with other disorders that exacerbate sexual compulsions, such as drug or alcohol abuse and depression, as well as social skills training.

Most convicted offenders are compelled to undergo treatment as a part of their probation or parole. In some states, those incarcerated undergo treatment in prison as their release date nears. There are far too few spaces in state prisons to treat all of those incarcerated for sexual abuse, and many of them begin intensive therapy just before release and continue treatment upon release.

At Bill Ford's Mustardseed, where most clients are sent by the courts as a part of probation or parole, Ford and his staff use cognitive behavior therapy to help clients recognize the thoughts and feelings that lead to deviant behavior, to take responsibility for their actions, and to learn how to control their urges and impulses. This process is the most common approach to treating sexual abusers, along with medication if necessary. A typical treatment program lasts two years. "If a person is living a reasonable lifestyle where they have a family, job, kids, the idea of anything interrupting that, such as jail, having to disclose to the family and public, is enough to nip it in the bud," Ford says. Some offenders lose ground and, based on Ford's recommendations to a parole or probation officer, they have to start the program over. "I have one guy who's been with me for three years. He had acted out before under the influence. He relapses on alcohol, loses his job," Ford says, noting that "relapse" in this case means returning to behavior patterns that once led to abuse, though not necessarily the abuse itself. "He talks to me, starts to readjust to the problem, and relapses again." For those who consistently relapse or who he determines are at very high risk of reoffending, Ford says, he recommends that they go back to prison.

Because there is no cure for sexual behavior disorders, experts are cautious about the degree of success of treatment. It's important to note that sexual offenders differ in how they approach victims, the factors that lead to abusive behavior, and the behavior itself. They also differ in terms of whether they are able to understand and take responsibility for their behavior. So they represent different levels of risk to society and warrant different types of response. But whatever their level of compulsion and risk, like drug addicts or alcoholics, sexual predators are considered recovering abusers who can lapse without proper intervention and support. But by combining treatment with supervision, studies have shown, many sexual abusers are less likely to reoffend.[13]

Scott Matson, a research associate at the Silver Spring, Maryland, Center for Sex Offender Management, which provides technical support to those who treat and manage offenders, says the issue is not whether offenders should be released from prison, but whether they are prepared to function in society.[14] "It's the question facing the entire criminal justice system," he says. "Do you ostracize all criminals forever, or bring them back into the fold?"

Matson compared doing time with doing a version of time and treatment: "If an individual does fifteen years without treatment, they can simply be released, and the criminal justice system will have no control over them," he says. "You may be able to keep tabs on them, but it's not conducive to rehabilitation. There is a push to begin as soon as the offender is incarcerated to prepare them to reenter the community. There are risk assessments, drug and alcohol abuse treatment. We build a treatment plan around this information and move to provide services like job skills training."

Recognizing that isolation is a major risk factor for sexual offenders, Matson says, many systems even require that offenders identify supports in their community—a church, a mentor, friends, or family members, even a boss or a coworker—before they are released. "Nobody's watching these guys daily," he says. "So the supervision and treatment are critical."

This is why the appropriate response to sexual abuse within our families is the same as if the crime is committed by a stranger off the street: Report it to the authorities, get the offender in the system, and seek help for the survivor and others who have been hurt. As Brenda, the Ohio mother, saw it, those were her only options.

ONE MOTHER'S RESPONSE TO ABUSE

When Brenda learned of her husband's abuse of her daughter, she knew immediately that it was a problem that was too big for her to handle alone. She knew because she had once worked as a secretary in a social services department and was aware of cases involving children who suffered physical, emotional, and sexual abuse. She knew that Charles had committed a crime, that she needed to get her children away from him and get the police involved. And she knew that Karla and her other children needed professional counseling. She also knew that Charles needed help, too. But even Brenda's professional knowledge could not prepare her for all that she and her family would experience.

It was 1992, and many supports like victim advocates—trained professionals who walk children and nonoffending parents or caregivers through the legal process—were just becoming common. Today these supports are standard in most abuse cases. Because she had once worked in social services, Brenda was surprised by the antagonism she faced when she entered the system as a client. As a mother and a wife, Brenda struggled with many complicated emotions and issues: She was horrified that her children were in danger, and she was consumed with guilt that she had not protected her daughter. She felt hurt and betrayed by her husband but still loved him, and she was afraid of facing the future alone.

It is a testament to Brenda's awareness and conviction that she was doing the right thing—for her children and for her husband—that she turned her husband in. Though she was far from perfect in responding to her husband, as her daughter describes, she managed to bring her family through a wrenching process. Their experience is an example of what happens in those rare situations when a parent believes the child and follows the advice of the experts.

KARLA'S (AND HER PARENTS') STORY: "EVERYTHING CHANGED"

Like life, this family's story is not so simple. It is a complex web of varying emotions and recollections. In the hopes of helping others in similar situations, Brenda, Karla's mother, wrote to me offering to share her experience. I asked Brenda to ask Karla, who was nineteen at the time, and Brenda's husband, Charles, forty-two, if they would also talk with me. When each said yes, I went to Ohio and met with Brenda and Karla separately. Then I went to the prison, where I spoke with Charles. As often happens when there are different perspectives on an incident or a situation, some key details conflict. In this case, there is one critical detail: Charles is adamant that the abuse lasted for less than two years, but Karla says it was more than four. The length of Charles's incarceration is perhaps the biggest indicator of the extent of the abuse: Scott Matson of the Center for Sex Offender Management says a seven-to-fifteen-year sentence is far longer than the national average of three to six years. Here are their accounts.

BRENDA (KARLA'S MOTHER)

When I first heard the news, I wanted to just quit on life. I had had a bad childhood living with domestic violence and alcoholism. I've always had to fight for everything in my life, and I didn't have any fight in me. I was giving up.

One of Karla's friends told Karla that she had been abused by a boyfriend of her mother's, and Karla then told the friend about her stepdad. The friend told Rochelle, my oldest daughter, and Rochelle told me. I don't remember a lot about that day, other than calling Karla into my bedroom. We sat down and I told her what her sister had told me. Then I asked her if it was true. We didn't really go into detail about what actually happened. That came later.

I don't know if I cried or what. I think I was in shock. But I believed Karla—I knew my daughters would never play a joke like that. I immediately packed up and moved me and the kids in with my mother. Then I called a friend who was an attorney.

I was a young mom. I'm thirty-eight now; I had Rochelle when I was sixteen. And then I had Karla at nineteen. They are now twenty-two and nineteen. I have two sons, one after Karla, by another man, and then one in '91, with Charles. My oldest son is eighteen, and the youngest is ten. The baby was one when his father went to prison in 1993. He will be fifteen or sixteen when his father gets out.

I haven't had the best luck with men. Karla's father got strung out on crack. He moved to another state when she was about three months old. Rochelle sees her father sometimes.

I met Charles at the production plant where we both worked. He was a manager and I was in human resources. I thought he was extremely bright. We dated for about a year before I even let him meet my kids. I was always like that—I didn't want my kids to meet anyone that I wasn't going to be serious about. He had kids, which made me feel comfortable. They were in another city. After we had dated awhile, he became my best friend.

We had a great relationship, and he seemed to like my kids. He was very supportive of my continuing my education—he had gone to college himself. He would help the kids with homework and do laundry and cook. Our sex life was good. He was giving, passionate, and attentive to my needs. He would send me roses to work "just because." I thought I had finally met the man of my dreams.

He was a disciplinarian, while I was more of the nurturer. My kids hated the fact that he was so strict. When we first started living together, it was a struggle. Hang up your coat. Don't play in the living room. Make up your bed. It was hard for them to go from little discipline to being disciplined to that degree. My first son, he didn't care for Charles too much. But he has always kept to himself.

Karla was about two when Charles came into our lives. She grew closest to him. She was what my family would call the bad child. Nobody wanted to take her anywhere. She had a lot of energy. Time-outs didn't work, spankings didn't work. I read a lot of parenting books to deal with her. But Charles always stuck up for her. He showed her more attention than the other kids. Whenever she asked for something, he would give it to her. But if my other daughter asked, he'd tell her no. He did favor Karla, but I always thought it was because Charles was really the only dad Karla knew.

The abuse lasted four years, from when she was six till about ten. The professionals believe that it may have even been longer. I know he had her perform oral sex, and that there was penetration. Karla never told me this—I learned it from the physical examination.

I had to tell his family. You hear about people taking sides, but my in-laws were very supportive. I'm close to his oldest sister, so I told her first. She fainted. His father cried. His sisters were very angry with him. They would often say to me that if it had been their daughter, they would have killed him. I've had several people say that to me, but where would that leave Karla, and where would that leave my other kids?

My own family had a difficult time, I think because I wasn't saying, "Hang him, castrate him." I was saying, "Yes, I want him to be incarcerated, but just don't throw him in there. Get him some help."

I know I did the right thing, but I struggled with it. I had just had the baby, I was working and going to school. We didn't have a lot of money but we were comfortable. I was worried about how I was going to make it with four kids on my own.

I blamed myself a lot. My question was always, "Brenda, how do you lay next to a man, sleep with a man every day, and not see what was going on? Did you ever get a feeling that something was wrong?" And I said no, 'cause Karla needed a dad. I didn't see their relationship as being unnatural. Everyone says you should know. But I didn't.

Charles and I cried a lot. I was so angry at him. But I never hated him because I don't believe in hate. I would ask him why over and over, and he would just say, "I don't know, I don't know." Once he was in jail he said that he had been abused himself by a family member or something like that. But I don't know why he would take it out on Karla.

One of the things that came up in therapy was why Karla? Why not the other kids? And I believe it was because Karla was needy, and he was able to provide her with the attention and protection, and to manipulate her.

When I called my friend the lawyer, she recommended that I contact the county children's services. They told me to bring the kids to their office. And then they interviewed each of them separately. I couldn't be present during the interviews. After that there were several investigations and meetings with detectives. Charles had moved out and stayed with a friend. Eventually he went in and was arrested.

During the beginning, my lawyer told me that they were thinking of bringing me up on charges too. But the lawyer told them that no, I came to them. It floored me. I thought that if I went to an agency for help, I would get help. This was so unfair. I really started to question myself. Did I know about it? Were there signs that I didn't want to see? And I became very careful about what I was saying, because I thought they were going to take my kids away.

The caseworkers were two White females. The first one was young—right out of college. They ordered that my kids stay with my mother. They were with her about three months. And that's when I thought about suicide. I had lived with domestic violence on my mom—it was her boyfriend. And here I try to fix this and have my kids separated from me? I just plummeted. But my Lord and Savior stepped in and told me no. I came to see that it was best that they were with her, because emotionally I was a wreck, and I needed time to get myself back up.

I think we all went through a healing process, with all that hurt and the anger. We did individual and family therapy, which helped Karla a lot. It helped her to understand that she did not do anything wrong. That he was taking advantage of her and using his power over her. She said he never threatened, and he didn't need to, because he was such a strong figure in her life. And that's what I want her to understand. Because she once said to me that she wished she had never said anything.

My concern has always been, "How am I going to help my kids?" For my oldest daughter, one of the things that came up was why had her sister been singled out and not her? But she was also glad that this was out in the open and being dealt with. And of course in therapy I did a lot of talking about how did I choose a man like this? And I had to go back and work on my own stuff. Because I saw how Charles was able to take advantage—roses just because.

One of the things I learned from therapy was about Karla's acting out. She did very well until she went to high school, then she just flipped. She always had this smiling face, and you would never have thought that anything was wrong. But then she would be violent toward other people. We could start out having a good day, and by the afternoon, the school would be calling and I'd have to go get her.

And then she would say that she'd had a nightmare and it was bothering her. Now how could I get on her case, knowing what probably provoked the nightmare?

I worried about my other children because so much attention was given to Karla. There was a lot of jealousy. The other kids would say, "Why does Karla get to get away with things?" And I would try to explain, "You may not see me chastise or discipline her, but know that I have. I'm not going to announce it to you because that's not your concern. Know that I'm dealing with it."

I write to Charles sometimes. Usually about what's going on with the kids, what's going on with me, and whatever I'm feeling that day. It used to be all the anger at first. I'd just totally blast him. Especially when Karla was acting out. Now I send pictures of when our youngest son is involved in events. And pictures of Karla's two kids, my granddaughter and grandson.

We're still married, but I've been trying to get a divorce for about a year now. I've told Charles that I'm working with an attorney. I always knew that I would get a divorce, but I haven't been in a hurry. One of my issues was the money for getting it done.

I wanted reunification at first. For all of us, if he could be helped. But I don't feel that way today. I could not lay down with him again and be his wife. I would feel like, "You did the same things with my daughter that you did with me." And I would wonder, "Are you thinking about my daughter when you're with me?" And I don't want to get into that. Then the other aspect is he wouldn't come to the relationship as an equal. I'd have something over him.

I still love him. He's still my best friend. It's not easy to admit, but it's the truth. I don't know if it's because of how I was raised or just that I once worked in the helping field, but I feel that when people are sick they can get help and they can change. I don't think that I'm betraying Karla by feeling that way. Because I believe that I did everything I could, once I found out, to protect her. And then I focused on helping her.

Karla's trying to move on with her life. It's going to take some time for her to get back on track. She's now a mother of two and so far she's doing a good job. The oldest is two, the other is about six months. She's working and I hope she goes back to finish high school.

But I worry about her kids. I'm always looking for signs. I'm always questioning Karla and who's around her.

She had said a long time ago that she was glad that Charles went to jail, rightfully so. I think that really has helped with her healing. She's written to him, and she will talk to him. But she's never wanted to go and visit him. I know she wants him to get out because of her youngest brother, she says, but she doesn't want to be around him.

We don't expect him to get out until 2006. He was already denied parole—Charles said somebody on the parole board told him he would not get out until Karla turned twenty-one. And then they told him, "When you do get out, I hope she blows your brains out."

Last year, I told my youngest son about his dad. Not in detail, but I said something like, "Remember when Mommy used to talk to you about good touches and bad touches? Well, your dad, he used bad touches on Karla. And that's why he has been in prison so long." He cries sometimes for his dad. It's tough.

To this day, I still don't have the answers. But I know that Karla has come through this and has received salvation through this. I'm so proud of the strides she has made. She is so strong. I know she is special and that God keeps His hand on her. For whatever reason, He made sure that we had the strength we needed to get through it.

We were a churchgoing family. And it's interesting, because earlier that year Charles got saved. It was about the time the abuse stopped. When I found out about it, I turned to the pastor, who was also my uncle, the same person who baptized me and married me. He was very supportive. I would often go to him for prayer—to pray with me and for me.

So Charles was a member of the church who disappeared. And I did too, eventually. One of the reasons was I didn't want to go through having to explain why he wasn't there. I went to another church, but I still stay in touch with my uncle.

At first I was mad at God. I would say to God, "Why not the family that was two streets over and on the corner?" I had believed that if you are under God's grace, that you're protected from harm. And that was a rude awakening. I stopped going to church altogether for a while. I started writing letters to God about what I was going through or what I was feeling. And still I had my relationship with Him.

I've been journaling since I was sixteen. Saved all of them. In my journal, here's the first thing that I wrote about this whole experience:

> I was advised by my attorney not to confront Charles. Well a couple of days went by and I couldn't contain this awful knowledge any longer. I confronted him, and of course he denied it. I could tell by the way his voice cracked when I let him know that I knew what he had been doing to Karla—I knew he was lying. After I told him that Karla had no reason to lie, he finally admitted some things. I felt so confused, hurt and in disbelief. I had finally found a decent man with strong family values and ties. Someone who thought I was pretty and would move the world for me if I asked him to. I felt so safe, so secure, so loved. Now my home has come tumbling down around me. There is no more security, nowhere to lay my head on his chest and know that everything is going—

I couldn't finish the sentence. Then I started to write about my youngest son—our son—and about how I needed to be sure to give him love and happiness.

CHARLES (KARLA'S STEPFATHER)

I couldn't tell you how it started. It was so gradual, I really didn't notice until it became a full-blown deal. I was always very fatherly with my children. I always hugged them, I always kissed them, I always told them I loved them, and I always wrestled with them and played with them. The sexual abuse was totally out of character. My character was about family.

Karla was always up under me. I would be sitting on the couch and she would come and crawl up in my arms and watch TV, or we would get to playing. She was a little tomboy. I would wrestle and fight and box with her. And during these times of, I guess, intimate father-daughter type relationships, it became more of a fondling type of play between me and the daughter. Initially, it was touching, sort of, laughing, playing, experimenting. Gradually it built up to actual sexual contact. I rubbed her. There was no penetration, but rubbing of the vagina, rubbing of the penis, oral sex, stuff like that.

She never said no. There was no coercion. I truly believe that she thought, "If Charles says this is okay, then this is okay." Karla was always getting into trouble, and it was always me that came to her rescue. So when I started sexually abusing her, I think she was under the assumption, "It just has to be okay, because Charles wouldn't hurt me."

It wasn't just that I had a sexual attraction. It could have been stress, work. It could have been drugs. I had started doing crack a lot. I never claimed that that was to blame for my crime—the court records show that. But I became more dependent on drugs and alcohol as a way to cover up my assault and depression. I distanced myself from positive friends and coworkers. I blamed my problems on my wife. And with the drugs and with the pressure, I lost my sense of morals. I had forgotten who I was and what my purpose was.

What led me to that? Stress, disappointment. Here I am making nice money, a nice job, but yet I started getting denied a lot of things. I wanted to buy a house in a nice neighborhood and they started denying me. I took on more responsibility at work, started stretching myself too thin. I stopped doing things that I enjoyed: running, playing racquetball, tennis. I spent more time drinking and hanging around with the wrong individuals. I had done cocaine before, but it was periodically, maybe on a holiday. I got to where I was doing it every weekend and then through the week. A fifth of liquor once lasted me a month or two. It began lasting me two or three days.

So I started blaming other people for things that were happening to me. I used to blame Brenda for spending money, but looking back, I was spending $200 a day on cocaine.

Brenda was angry with me. And the more angry she got, the more I blamed her for messing around. But she wasn't. We started distancing ourselves, and I think that kind of sent me to my daughter. Because Karla started becoming my friend. She would always come up to me, when I would be down, with a smile, a hug and kiss. That's what I would look for from Brenda. My counselor called it role-changing. I saw Karla as the person that I would confide in. Basically my wife.

She was about nine when it started. I know everybody was saying it happened for like five or six years. But Karla was probably about five when Brenda and I moved in together. And we were living together a couple of years before it actually started, so she had to have been like eight or nine.

When Brenda confronted me, I knew there was nothing I could say. It was kind of like I had traded in my marriage, my relationship, not just her trust, but the trust of my entire family. I was devastated. I wouldn't eat and constantly would get sick. A couple of times I would take showers—and I've got scars on my body—I would just take a brush and scrub myself, because I felt so, I don't know, dirty. I wanted to just get that person out of me. It was like I was trying to scrub myself clean.

Brenda and I were always best friends. I knew she was the one because she was very outgoing, and she had all the qualities that I liked in a woman—culturally diverse, adventurous, willing to try new things. She was very open, and somebody that I could trust. She had three kids when I met her. And I had two. It was a lot to take on, but I was blessed with a good job—they paid me very good. I was higher up in the organization. So to take on the responsibility of extra children was never a problem.

I grew up in a family of humanitarians. They were always helping somebody out. We were teased a lot about being upper-middle-class. Many people would call us the Cosbys. My parents sent me and my older three sisters to college. I'm currently taking correspondence courses in business and economics.

My parents were very open, very honest, very blunt. I think that's where me and my sisters get it from. Even though we love each other, if you're wrong, we're going to tell you you're wrong. Even in crisis, my parents had a way of helping us see there were lessons to learn from what happened.

I'm the baby of our family, and the only boy. It was like having four mothers. I could talk to all of them. When they found out that I had gotten a young lady pregnant, they all came to me saying, "Why didn't you use protection?" I was twenty when I had my first kids. They're by two different mothers, ten days apart.

My sisters were very angry about what I did to Karla. They've got kids. I had moved out of the house and was living with my friend, and my sisters sent word to keep my distance. The message went, "We will hurt you right now." That's understandable. Because they got the impression that I was denying this. But from the beginning, I never denied it. My father had to bring them around. We had a family meeting, where I told them what happened. And I think that as long as they saw progress in me, they were willing to help.

This is actually how I got incarcerated: It was about me being open to go and tell somebody, "Hey, I did this, and I want some advice." The abuse had been going on for about a year, maybe a year and a half, when one day I was sitting on the couch—I was at home by myself and the kids were outside playing, and Karla came in and crawled up on me and started putting her hands down in my pants. I grabbed her hands and I held on to her so tight that she screamed that I was holding her too tight. I think that scared her.

She scared me because she had conditioned herself that when she comes in the house and I'm in there by myself and she can lay on me, and it's okay to reach in my pants. [*He pauses.*] I guess in a way I conditioned her—not intentionally, but yeah, I conditioned her to say that, whenever we're alone, you can do this.

The next month, I called this counselor, a psychologist who was experienced with sexual abuse. He asked if I had reported it yet, and I said no. At that time, I didn't know that the daughter had gone to her mother and they had reported it. So when my counselor called to report it, he said they already had a warrant for my arrest.

I was never really arrested. The sheriff came up to my house and left a calling card. He said, "Hey, we've got a warrant for your arrest; you need to get with your attorney." So I went down to the office. From the time that Brenda reported it to the first hearing, it was almost two years.

During that time I was still working. I told my immediate supervisor what had happened. He was in disbelief. At my company, in my department, I was next in line after him. These guys respected me. It was like a family outside of a family. So I felt like I let them down also.

During the hearings I was staying with my friend and going to sexual abuse classes and seeing the counselor. And I was addressing my drug habit. I stopped doing drugs and I started getting back to the person that I was.

In counseling I had started to learn a lot about what I did, and how this hurt everybody. When I realized the magnitude of this, it just blew me away. I felt hurt, shamed, and disgusted within myself. I could never see myself hurting someone, especially someone I love. I'm not a violent person.

And I realized that I was molested at about four or five. My older sisters had girlfriends who used to stay the night, and they used to sneak in the bathroom with me. They were all teenagers. We used to have a couple of babysitters who used to let me lay on them and play with them. I never thought of that as being molested. I always thought it was just being sneaky. The counselor told me that it was being molested.

Since I've been incarcerated they have denied me any type of rehabilitation. I'm on the waiting list for treatment. People who come in with flat time get priority. Flat time is when somebody gets, say, five years, where I'm doing seven to fifteen. I can do anywhere from seven years to the maximum fifteen. I've done eight so far, and the parole board has already denied me once. If somebody is only going to do five, they'll get them into treatment first. And I'll have to wait. Most likely, I will have to do all fifteen years before I get considered.

The first time I called home from prison they said, "Wait a minute, somebody here is dying to talk to you," and it was Karla. And I think I was quiet the whole time and just let her talk. She asked me if I was doing okay and if anybody was bothering me or anything like that, and I told her no. I think she was more worried about me. And I told her, "Don't worry about me." I tried to let her know, "I'm here if you ever need anything. If you want to get your frustration out on me, write me a bad letter, cuss me out all day long, that's what I'm here for." I've apologized to her, so many times. I've apologized to the whole family.

I told them I am sorry, and that I was wrong, face-to-face, on the phone, letters, cards. I know they hate what I did. I'm ashamed for letting down the family.

I told my youngest son too. I tried to keep it in language that he would understand. I would say, "I touched her inappropriately." And he would say, "What do you mean by inappropriate?" "I touched her in places where people shouldn't touch." And he would say, "In her private place?" I'd say, "Exactly."

I know Karla's been traumatized by what has happened. I was probably the only person outside of her mother that she actually trusted and loved. And I destroyed that. I know that if I had never done this, Karla would never have gotten pregnant at an early age. I know she had sleeping disorders. I know that when she went to high school they said that she would skip school and go have sex with boys. Since she's kind of like gotten a little older, she's kind of matured. But I can tell in her letters that she's going through some problems now.

I must say that I don't truly understand the impact of my crime on Karla. Do I want to understand, to have empathy? Yes, I do. I also thought about what I could do to help prevent others from making the same mistake. They should admit they were wrong immediately. Don't try to hide it behind religion or keep it in the family secret closet. That will only make the victim feel it was their fault. Or worse, begin a cycle of sexual abuse for the victim. Accept the punishment.

I think my sentence is just. But not compared to others. Just because I'm not a politician or a Catholic priest, their sentences should be no different. But prison is nothing. It will be over one day. I will incarcerate myself for the rest of my life. I will always punish myself for what I did. When I get out, I don't know what kind of relationship I'm going to have with anyone in my family. There are many—if not all—who would rather not be associated with me. I understand.

A lot of people are, I guess, ashamed to admit or to talk about their problems or what they have done. Yeah, I'm ashamed of what I've done, but I'm not ashamed to talk about it, because I know it would never happen again.

KARLA

I'm nineteen, but people say I act about thirty. Maybe it's the kids. I would describe myself as responsible, strong, giving, loving.

I was a middle child for a long time, and I was always in trouble. I was misunderstood. I know I had a lot of energy. I'd do things like put fingernail polish on the wall, then stick paper to it, or break my mom's elephants, or get into the fridge at night. My sister was considered the good one. She got all the attention for being good. My brother was always good too. I didn't care. I didn't bond with my sister when I was younger. I remember being by myself a lot.

I was about five or six when Mom married Charles. But the abuse started before they got married. I remember going to his apartment—my aunt would watch us over there. Sometimes Charles and I would be there by ourselves. He started putting me on his lap at his apartment. He went on to touching me and oral sex. He never entered me, though.

It would often happen in his car, too. He'd say, "Let's go to the store," and then he'd do it—he'd have me perform oral sex while he was driving. Charles doesn't think it was longer than a year or so, but he did things that he may not consider abuse.

I'd say it was physical abuse too. Charles would beat us. He hit my sister upside the head for staying out too late. He beat us with an extension cord, until my mom stood up against that. I felt afraid of him.

I remember crying when they got married.

When I was about ten, my friend told me that her mom's boyfriend touched her one time. After she told me her story I told her mine. Later my friend said her story was made up.

I remember my mom calling me upstairs and asking me if it was true. I said yes. I remember me sitting in a room, and a lot of people around me, asking me all kinds of questions.

The next thing I knew we were at my grandmother's house.

Before Charles went to jail, my mother would let him come back to the house to visit. He didn't stay around, but I was upset about that. I felt like she was taking his side. My sister was mad, and my grandmother, too.

When my sister told, I was scared that Charles would beat me, or that my mom would think I was lying. I always remember being angry at my real father, thinking that none of this would have happened if he didn't leave me. I didn't have a man to love me, and I thought this was the way a father loves a daughter. I didn't realize how bad it was until I went to counseling.

I was never angry at my sister for telling my mother. I never talked about it with her. I figured she knew enough, and my brother was too young. But I felt responsible for what was happening. We moved out of the house I grew up in. Charles went to jail. My brother lost a father. It took a lot of counseling to teach me that I wasn't responsible.

I started counseling when I was about eleven. I did it for two years—first group, then one-on-one. I liked group better, because it made me feel as if I wasn't alone. Everybody had been through the same kind of thing. The therapist was White, and most in the group were White. These White women wanted me to draw a picture of Charles and punch it on a punching bag. That felt comfortable, but it didn't make much sense to me.

I was angry at myself for a long time. So much changed, everything changed when Mom found out about Charles. I thought I'd caused it. Counseling helped me see that it wasn't my fault. It was Charles's fault.

I'm so glad my mom believed me. I thought she'd say I was a liar. I thought Mom would stop loving me if I told her.

His side of the family—it felt different. It felt like it was my fault. It made me sad.

I thought my aunts would stop loving me for sending their brother to jail. It was something I imagined, because I know I have their support. I thought my cousins didn't like me. I thought that they thought I was a liar. It's OK to see them, but when we get together, it's not like it used to be.

Looking back, I'd say my sexuality was definitely affected. I became sexually active at fourteen—just because I knew about sex. Not just knowing, but I knew firsthand what to do. I'd been taught. I had sexual urges too, before I was fourteen.

I also acted out. I had sex with many boys—boys from school, boys I'd meet on the street. If my mother knew, she'd probably be very surprised.

It wasn't uncomfortable to have sex, but I can't say I knew what intimacy was. I felt as if a guy wanted sex, I just had to give it to them no matter what. Even if I didn't want to. After sex was over, there was no love. I felt used, dirty, just really nasty.

One time I skipped school and went with some guys to another guy's house. They got the idea that I would have sex with all ten of them. They started taking off my clothes. I just grabbed my stuff and ran. I went to school and told what happened. They sent me to a support group. Nothing happened to the boys.

When I was sixteen, I went into foster care. My mom couldn't handle me. I was running away, not listening, out of control. They took me from my home, and that's when I found out I was pregnant.

The father of my daughter—I feel like I'm still waiting for him to grow up. I'd seen him for three years. We still stay in touch, and he takes my daughter sometimes. But there's no chance of us getting together.

The father of my son, Paul—he's been very helpful. We're the same age. We really clicked. He's a wonderful father—he's much more sensitive than the men I've known. He was a virgin when we met—I'd never had any experience like that. This was so new to me. He didn't want me physically—he loved me. I never knew how that felt before. I was more used to guys just wanting sex. I was in love. We've gotten engaged. I don't know if I'll get married right now. There's so much I want to do.

I told Paul about being abused. Charles had sent this birthday card, and Paul asked who was Charles. I told him it was my stepfather, who was in jail. Paul asked why he was in jail, and I told him for molesting me. He was okay with it. He told me about things in his family too.

I send letters to Charles sometimes. In one of them, I asked if he would pay for the wedding. He said yes—anything I needed.

I'm not angry and I'm not sad. He apologized and I don't hate him. But when he gets out, I don't want to see him. There was a time when he told my mother that I would come to him, and that I started it. That really bothers me. How could I go to him to do what he did to me?

My sister has taken care of me. She lives with me and helps with the kids. My mother was very helpful. She helped me forgive Charles. She said God had already forgiven him—why couldn't we?

I feel like I've come a long way, but I could be so much more if I didn't start having babies. If this hadn't happened, I would have gotten my education. I've got two babies now, working on my GED. I feel I'm still waiting for my life to begin—the rest of my life.

FLAWS IN THE SYSTEM

The system that is set up to deal with child sexual abuse is far from perfect: bias, overwhelmed child protective services agencies, insensitivity to survivors, inconsistency in prosecution and sentencing. These flaws contribute to why people don't report cases to the authorities. But the system is improving. Most police departments now have advocates who can walk survivors through the legal process, as well as sensitivity training for officers responding to complaints. And experts remind us that the alternatives to reporting are far, far worse. The Rosa Parks Sexual Assault Crisis Center in Los Angeles, which serves primarily African American and Latina clients, is often the first place that people in the area turn to when they learn or suspect that a child has been sexually abused. Dr. Jeanne Hartsfield, who conducts initial interviews of clients, has seen mothers walk away once they hear that an abuser will be prosecuted. She tries to assure them that the most important thing to remember at such a stressful time is the safety of the child. "It's a big dilemma for many people, though it shouldn't be," she says. "Yes, a person might be found guilty, they might go to jail, and yes, it's a painful experience. But the child needs to feel safe, protected, cared about. The child should not have to go away with a sense of alienation and rejection that they will live with the rest of their lives."

In the center's counseling service for adult survivors, Hartsfield sees the other side of this coin: women who as children disclosed abuse to their families and were ignored, spanked, scolded, or told not to talk about it. "This impacts an overwhelming number of clients," she says. "They have tried to work out these issues on their own with their families. When they come to us they are desperate. Many of them have told me that the reason they never reported the abuse is that the family didn't believe them."

One major system flaw that experts point to is when allegations of sexual abuse are a part of separation or divorce proceedings. Eileen King, regional director for Justice for Children, a national advocacy organization that intervenes when agencies fail to protect kids, says that bias and inadequate information often lead family court judges to decide in favor of husbands seeking custody or unsupervised visitation. She argues that when child sexual abuse allegations arise, the criminal justice system courts should get involved. "Oftentimes, when abuse arises in separation cases, the assumption is that it's in response to a custody dispute and it is not taken seriously," she says. In family court proceedings, unlike criminal court, she says, the goal is often a ruling "in the best interest of the child," which may or may not have to do with the child's safety. For instance, a family court judge could decide that it is in the child's "best interest" to see both parents.

And, of course, there are ongoing debates about incarceration versus treatment of sexual abusers, and whether courts should hear from survivors on these issues. In some cases, depending on the severity of the abuse, survivors may indeed have a say in how the system responds to offenders. Solomon, a client for five years at Mustardseed, the Brooklyn counseling service for sexual abusers, was ordered to undergo treatment as part of his five years of probation. His crime: sexual abuse of his eleven-year-old stepdaughter, Janice, over the course of three months. At his sentencing hearing, Solomon's stepdaughter asked that he be sent to treatment instead of incarceration. He knows that her request helped to make all the difference in his punishment.

ONE MAN'S TREATMENT

Solomon, forty-five, is what Bill Ford calls one of his success stories. He has a regular job, is drug-free, and makes use of social support systems to stay on track. He still stops by Mustardseed to check in even though he is not required to, and Ford often has him address new groups of offenders or speak about his deviancy to probation and parole officers to help them better understand how sexual abusers operate.

He has not returned to his family's home and will not, he says. He does not think it would be in the best interest of his wife, Laura, who married him while he was on probation for sexually abusing her daughter, or in the best interest of the three younger girls they had together who are still living at home (Janice, who is eighteen, has now moved out). To give a sense of what happens when abusers undergo treatment, I thought it would be useful to hear briefly about Solomon's experiences and perspective on his sexual behavior disorder, and to contrast his with those of Charles, who is serving out his sentence with no treatment since being imprisoned in 1993:

"I was using my crack addiction as a crutch. If I wasn't high, I wouldn't do it, but if I wanted it, I'd get high first. I remember thinking sometimes that it wasn't as bad a crime because she wasn't my daughter. You know, that sick way of thinking. I would have her perform masturbation on me, or I would masturbate and have her watch. I would touch her, tell myself I was teaching her how to kiss. Once I had her sit in my lap and look at porno films. I performed oral sex on her. It got to the point where it was every day, if possible. It started scaring her. She'd say, 'This isn't right; you're supposed to be my father.' There were times that she would cry and I'd feel guilty as sin. I'd tell her that she could tell. I didn't have enough backbone to do it myself.

"I started giving her money. I'd tell her that her mother and I weren't getting along, so this was okay. I started telling her that when she decided that she wanted to have sex that I wanted to be the first one to put it in. That's what frightened the hell out of her."

When Janice told her mother, she immediately removed the children and called the police and sent Janice to therapy, Solomon says. Investigations and physical examinations showed that Janice was the only girl abused. At first Solomon denied abusing Janice, but later admitted it so she wouldn't have to testify. Initially, he was facing seven to fifteen years for molestation of a child. Janice and Laura spoke to a prosecutor in the district attorney's office. In private, Laura shared with the prosecutor what Solomon had told her long ago: that as a boy he had been abused by his mother and one of her friends. After a risk assessment, Solomon was directed to register with the state as a sex offender, to report to Mustardseed for mandatory counseling, and to get treatment for his drug addiction. He was also ordered not to have contact with any of his children during probation. He underwent daily therapy for the first year, then weekly group therapy sessions for the next four.

"I used to have to tell my story every day—we'd go around the room and say our name, age, and why we were there. I didn't want to talk about any of this. It would hurt hearing me tell a room full of guys that I molested my eleven-year-old. I didn't want to admit to people what I did. In therapy I learned what a good bullshit artist I was. At times I'd try to color things a certain way, but Bill would stop me in my tracks. He'd make me go back and really listen to myself and think about what I was saying. I finally learned how to think about what another person is feeling. I'm not as much of a selfish and self-centered bastard as I used to be."

It's been two years since his probation ended. Nearly every day he calls the children who still live at home. Occasionally he calls Janice. When he initially spoke with her, he thanked her for telling and reassured her that she did the right thing. And he apologized "for not knowing how to show her real love." He has told her that if she ever says she doesn't want to talk with him, he won't call. If he's ever in her company and she wants him to leave, he will. Whether she loves him or not, it's okay. Whatever she wants, he will accept. And he has accepted that his actions seven years ago will have consequences for the rest of his life.

"I gave up a relationship with a daughter that I may never get back," he says. "My wife allows me to see my kids, but I prefer to have someone else present. It bothers me because sometimes I'd just like to take my daughters out shopping or to a movie, but I have to keep a realistic look at things." Solomon equates his sex addiction to his drug addiction, and recalls his twelve-step training: "Truthfully, I have no intentions of picking up a drug ever again. But I don't know how I'll wake up feeling tomorrow. I have to treat this sex offense the same way. It's not that I don't trust myself. Actually I do—for today."

LEGAL REMEDIES FOR ADULT SURVIVORS

Adult survivors who want to legally challenge child sexual abusers have two routes: criminal prosecution and a civil suit. If you venture into this territory, tread carefully. Many survivors pursue legal remedies as a way to have their day in court. This course of action can be empowering, advocates and mental health experts say, but it can also be emotionally and physically draining. As one sexual abuse recovery expert writes: "For some survivors, a lawsuit is a public announcement of their intention to force the perpetrator to make amends for [his] actions; for others, it becomes another form of abuse."[15] Rhea Almeida of the Institute for Family Services describes one of her clients' experience with criminal prosecution: "She went to the prosecutor to press charges. Then she gave several statements. Then there were extended interviews over several months. It went on and on. She realized she had to prove her case to the prosecutor before they would move forward. Eventually she gave up." Attorneys take on cases that they can win, and sexual abuse cases stemming from years ago are not the most promising. "Many prosecutors are reluctant to take on sexual abuse cases unless they involve a child or unless the abuser still poses a risk to children" through work, religious, or volunteer activities, Almeida says. Knowing this shouldn't deter you from exploring legal redress; it should help you think realistically about how persuasive your case would be to a judge or a jury.

No matter how solid your case, do not pursue either remedy without giving careful thought to whether you are healed enough to recall and discuss publicly and in detail deeply personal and painful experiences. Don't expect that a guilty verdict will help you heal. Your first and best way to recover from trauma is through therapeutic means. Speak with a counselor and friend who can provide emotional support, and contact a local sexual assault crisis center to talk with someone who can help you explore which options might be best, based on your experiences.

Consider these questions before you pursue a legal challenge:

- What do you hope to gain by taking legal action?
- How do you want your abuser to be held accountable?
- How do you feel knowing your experiences will be shared in a public venue?
- How do you feel about your motives or character being questioned in a civil trial?
- How would you feel if your actions led some family members to turn against you?
- How would you feel if you do not win?
- Can you afford the time and emotional investment of a criminal or civil trial (either process can last for a year or longer)?
- What evidence do you have, beyond your word, that you were abused, that could persuade a judge or jury?

If you do decide to pursue legal action, know that each state has its own statute of limitation, or a limit on the time in which you can press criminal charges or file a civil complaint. In response to pressure from victims' rights organizations and to the emergence of survivors of sexual abuse by clergy, many states have extended their statutes in child sexual abuse cases. These extensions recognize that some survivors do not recall that they were abused until therapy or some other event triggers the memory many years later.[16] The "Help Yourself" section at the end of this chapter offers a few places to start for general information on statutes. For more details on the laws in your state, contact your local prosecutor's office regarding criminal statutes or an attorney regarding civil statutes.

Once you've considered your personal concerns and expectations and done your homework on your state's statute of limitations, you can decide whether to move forward. If you do, this general overview will give you a sense of what to expect from criminal or civil actions:[17]

Criminal Prosecution

In a criminal prosecution, the state charges that a person has committed a "crime against the state." You are considered a witness to the crime. The process works to prove the guilt or innocence of the defendant (the person charged), and the penalty is usually punishment by fine paid to the government, imprisonment, probation, or counseling. To pursue criminal prosecution, you make a report to the police, who then conduct an investigation. If they arrest and charge the person accused, they will turn over investigation results to the district attorney's office, which assigns a prosecuting attorney. The prosecutor then decides whether to prosecute. If not, the charges are dropped. If the prosecution goes forward, the state argues its case, with you testifying as a witness. You will likely be assigned a victim/witness advocate who can accompany you through the criminal justice process, or you can seek one on your own through a local rape crisis center or the National Organization for Victim Assistance (NOVA), www.trynova.org. More information is in the Resources section of this book.

Criminal cases are most often tried before a jury with a judge presiding. (If the case is brought against a juvenile, it will be tried by a judge.) The jury will be seeking to answer these questions: (1) Did a crime occur? (2) Did the defendant commit the crime?

In a criminal trial, the standard of proof is high: The state must convince a jury *beyond a reasonable doubt* that the person you accused did in fact commit the crime he or she has been charged with. That means that if there is a reasonable doubt, based on the evidence, the accused should not be convicted. Many cases of sexual abuse, especially those in which no physical evidence has been recorded or recovered (cuts, scratches, bruising, DNA from sperm), are very difficult to prove beyond a reasonable doubt. Perhaps that explains why Almeida's client felt as if she had to prove her case to the prosecutor.

Civil Suit

A civil suit aims to determine that the person accused is liable, or responsible, for injuries that you have sustained as a result of his or her crime. In a civil case, the aim is not to determine the guilt or innocence of the accused, or to incarcerate. If the court finds the person is liable, then the defendant is held accountable to the plaintiff (the person bringing the suit), and must pay monetary damages. You can file a civil suit even if your offender was found not guilty in a criminal trial. Survivors have sought payment for medical expenses, psychological counseling, recovery of lost wages, and "pain and suffering," among other things. The standard of proof in a civil case is by a *preponderance of the evidence,* meaning that you must prove that your claims are most likely true and that you were harmed by the actions of the defendant. To bring a civil suit, you should consult with an attorney. (The "Help Yourself" section at the end of this chapter lists several places to begin your search and helps you prepare for your meeting.) Be sure to discuss payment. Many attorneys will take a case on contingency, that is, they will take their payment out of any money you recover from the defendant if you win. They will have you sign a contract for representation, called a retainer agreement for their services, and may require some payment up front. After interviewing you and reviewing your information, the attorney will determine whether your case is worth pursuing. But you, too, should use your discussion as a chance to interview the attorney. Make sure you feel comfortable with the person and his or her manner; the attorney should seem to understand what you want to accomplish. You may want to consult more than one attorney to find a good fit. Unlike in a criminal case where the attorney represents the state, in a civil case your attorney represents you. This gives you much more control over the decisions shaping the case. Your attorney helps you decide whether to sue, accept a settlement offer, or go to trial. Some key points you should consider in civil actions:

- The defendant's attorney can request your personal and private documents related to the case, including mental or physical health records and diary or journal entries.
- The defendant may also countersue you. Defendants have been known to do this to harass or intimidate survivors into withdrawing their suits.
- Just because you win a judgment does not mean the defendant will pay. Some defendants do not or cannot pay judgments entered against them. You may find that, years after a verdict, you are still fighting for payment.

Whatever the outcome of a criminal or civil case, you can still seek monetary compensation from your state's crime victims compensation board. These programs are often subject to restrictions and limitations. While neither a criminal conviction nor a monetary award can make up for a traumatic experience, pursuing legal remedies can give you a measure of satisfaction and empowerment for challenging your offender and holding him accountable for his actions. The best thing you can do before pursuing these options is to learn the facts and laws in your state and get a realistic sense of the challenges you may face in pursuing legal remedies. With the support of friends and family, you can then determine what's best for you.

Legal redress is just one way of resolving a history of sexual abuse. I will explore other ways in the next chapter.

HELP YOURSELF

Legal Issues and Finding a Lawyer

Finding a lawyer is your first step in pursuing a civil case against a sexual abuser. You want someone you feel comfortable with, who works well with survivors, and who has successfully brought child sexual abuse cases, or at least has knowledge of victims law. Start with your local rape or sexual assault victim crisis center, your state sexual assault coalition (http://www. rainn.org/scasa.html), or your local chapter of the National Organization for Women (NOW). Here are some other resources:

The National Crime Victim Bar Association (2000 M Street, NW, Suite 480, Washington, DC 20036; 800-FYI-CALL, (202) 467-8753; www. victimbar.org) is a network of attorneys and other professionals that provides referrals to local attorneys in victim-related litigation. The NCVBA is an affiliate of the National Center for Victims of Crime. E-mail victimbar@ ncvc.org.

Justice for Children (733 15th Street NW, Suite 214, Washington, DC 20005; (202) 462-4688; www.jfcadvocacy.org) maintains a lawyers referral list by state.

The **Martindale-Hubbell Lawyer Locator**, www.martindale.com, is the online version of the advertising directory for lawyers. You can search by geographical area, name, and specialty, among other options.

Your state's bar association may have a referral service. You can find state affiliates through the national organizations, the **American Bar Association**, www.abanet.org, or the **National Bar Association**, the organization of African American attorneys, www.nationalbar.org.

Preparing for the Attorney

From the beginning, your attorney will want to determine whether your evidence will convince a judge or jury of a defendant's crime or responsibility for your injury. Be as cooperative as you can. And be prepared to answer these questions:[18]

- Dates and times of the criminal or damaging events
- Location of events, including addresses and description of the premises
- Witnesses
- How the offender gained access to you
- Whether a police report was ever filed, and if so, identification of the detective or officer on the case, the complaint or report number, and statements taken as part of the investigation
- Whether there was ever or is a criminal case, and if so, the name of the prosecutor and the status of the case
- The nature of your relationship to the offender, the offender's name, address, date of birth, and Social Security number, employment information, and any information about the offender's assets and insurance coverage
- A physical description of the offender, including any identifying features
- The degree of physical, emotional, and psychological injuries, and the extent and cost of anticipated treatment
- Identification of the hospital, clinic, or other source of medical care related to your abuse
- Lost amount of time from work, lost wages, disability insurance

Statutes of Limitations

The Web sites below include extensive information on criminal and civil statutes of limitations in sexual abuse cases. These resources are for your general reference only; consult a local attorney or prosecutor's office, because the laws in your state may have changed.

The **National Center for Victims of Crime** has information on extensions of criminal and civil statutes: www.ncvc.org/gethelp/statutes-oflimitations/index.html.

RAINN, the Rape, Assault and Incest National Network, includes a state-by-state list of criminal statutes at http://www.rainn.org/statutes-oflimitationcrim.html.

You can also get state-by-state information at www.smith-lawfirm.com, an informative Web site maintained by **Susan Smith**, a Hartford, Connecticut, attorney specializing in family law and sexual abuse cases.

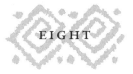

EIGHT

Reconciliation . . . and Moving On

3/16/96 9:20 P.M.
I spent the weekend in Charlotte. Went to Aunt _____'s for the first time since June '92. That's when I had confronted _____ about what he did to me as a child. I was indeed very uncomfortable. . . . I wonder if she knew anymore about the family secret. I felt she did. At least his version. . . . Home doesn't feel like home anymore. Things have changed. People have changed. . . . It's really got me thinking I should move away from family. I feel like just walking away—and not looking back.

—GAIL, thirty-seven, who was abused by her stepfather
and uncle from age nine to sixteen

GAIL, A COUNSELOR AT A NORTH CAROLINA SEXUAL ASSAULT CRISIS center, wrote the above entry in her journal. Gail, who was repeatedly abused by her stepfather and uncle from age nine to sixteen, had become so conditioned to sex by the adults' assaults that she propositioned a brother and her teenage cousins. They eagerly accepted. "At one point," she told me, "I was having sex with everybody."

When she was fourteen, at the urging of a girlfriend she'd confided in, Gail wrote her mother a note explaining that her stepfather was "touching her" under the covers at night. Gail had seen him beat her mother and had narrowly escaped beatings herself, so she hoped her disclosure would force him out of their lives. But Gail did not tell about her uncle, who had raped her. His wife, Gail's aunt, was her favorite. She worried about breaking her heart.

It should come as no surprise that Gail did not reveal the identities of both abusers. Adult survivors can probably understand her struggle to find a way to coexist with the people who abused her and the people she loved. Sometimes those people are one and the same. For many, the biggest fear of disclosing abuse is that they will disrupt or lose their family. As Karla said in Chapter 7, "everything changed" once her secret came out.

Their concerns are understandable. Culturally, African Americans hold dear the notion of family; our reverence stems not only from the significance our African ancestors placed on kin and clan, but also from the fact that our bonds were once so fragile. In times of slavery our great-great-great-grands could only watch helplessly as their children were sold and dragged off to points unknown. After the Civil War and Emancipation, our families were still dispersed as many left for big cities in search of jobs and better opportunities. Many African Americans place family above everything, and many survivors simply are unwilling to risk those cherished family connections. In fact, some will settle for a life of superficial or inequitable ties rather than none at all.

Janet Davis, the senior clinical social worker at the Northside Center for Children, a Harlem community mental health center for adults as well as kids, says that in her twenty years of individual, family, and group counseling, about 50 percent of the clients she has seen have divulged a history of sexual abuse—most often by family members. But not one has pressed charges or filed a civil suit against an abuser.

Why? Lack of money and knowledge of and access to legal services, she says. But more often, clients who come to her are more focused on making themselves—and their families—whole. "I don't think our people come from the perspective that they can take someone to court," she says. "They're trying to get better."

This chapter has been the most difficult part of my book to write because there are no easy answers to the question of how you find healing and keep—or sever—family connections. Or the question of whether it is healthy to stay connected at all. The experts tell us what we should do, but ultimately each of us must decide what's best. What I have learned, both personally and in my interviews, is that once they acknowledge and disclose the abuse, many survivors find that they must renegotiate relationships in their families. That renegotiation depends on many factors, among them:

- Your relationship to the abuser
- The length and severity of the abuse
- The amount of work you've done to heal
- The degree of support you receive from family members
- How often you interact with family members

- The strength of support systems outside of your family
- Your faith or spiritual foundation

CAN YOU BE A FAMILY AGAIN?

While most therapists don't push clients to leave their families, they do help them renegotiate relationships so they are in a position of power. Davis at first warns survivors that it is not their responsibility to hold their family together. Often a survivor has so much work to do on self that it is too difficult to bring others along too. After she sees a client making progress, Davis will introduce the idea of bringing other family members to therapy. She offers a code of conduct to help guide discussions (see the "Help Yourself" section at the end of this chapter).

Maelinda Turner, the San Francisco social worker, helps survivors understand the costs of keeping quiet to keep the peace. "Many would rather live in the illusion that everything is okay," Turner says. "The thinking is that they've already lost so much, they are just not willing to give that up. I've had many people say, 'Well, my parents are getting old.' That has the effect of putting the needs of the family above your needs."

Rhea Almeida, whose Institute for Family Services in New Jersey serves a large group of domestic violence as well as sexual abuse survivors, helps clients put themselves first. "Our motto is not that we keep families together," she says. "We say to them that you need to deal with the oppression, the power issues in the family, and then you decide whether you can stay or whether the family can stay together, rather than saying, 'Let's keep this family together no matter what.' If you can work it out, terrific. If not, tough."

That's a harsh reality for many survivors. While you may not have to walk away, as Gail contemplated in her journal, can you ever be a family again? It is a question that I returned to time and again as I interviewed survivors and as I considered my own circumstances. This answer, too, is not so simple. "You can continue being a family, but just not the same family you were," explains Dorothy Cunningham, the New York psychoanalyst. If you decide to remain a part of your family, you must do so on your own terms.

Many survivors are simply seeking a validation that the abuse happened and an acknowledgment of their pain. Some seek an apology. Some seek amends. But as we know, not everybody gets the response they are looking for. Abusers deny, parents move on, family members say, "Get over it." Many survivors find themselves frustrated and angry, waiting for words of comfort that may never come. Experts say that kind of thinking is giving others power to determine your happiness.

What you must do, they say, is decide how you move on, regardless of what others say or do. And how you move on depends on how you resolve your history of abuse.

FINDING RESOLUTION

Resolution—accepting that sexual abuse is a part of your past, but determining that it does not have to be a part of your future—is a critical part of the healing process. It is the point at which you can put the abuse into the larger context of your life, Almeida says. "Not just the events of physical violation," she says, "but the other aspects of resilience in your life that you can celebrate—that are your backbone. It's when the focus moves from the trauma to how you were able to survive." When she leads her group therapy sessions, she sees movement toward resolution when clients can ask one another, "When he was raping you, who in your life was being helpful to you?"

Resolution is when the fear, the anger, the memories, the flashbacks no longer affect how you navigate your relationships. It is when you can function at work without being overwhelmed. Or if you don't enjoy the work you do, you are looking for other work. When you are resolved, you hold the power to determine your own happiness, and you can move forward with your life regardless of the response from others.

For me, resolution meant honoring my own level of comfort, even if that meant that others in my family were uncomfortable. When I first wrote about my sexual abuse in *Essence,* I received hundreds of letters and e-mails from people as far away as Africa and Europe about how brave I was for tackling an issue that few want to talk about. But back at home, one relative called me selfish for embarrassing everyone and healing myself "at the expense of the family." Initially, that criticism from one so close overshadowed all the encouraging words from strangers. It was something I had to explore so I could move forward. I never felt brave baring my most vulnerable self to millions of readers; I wrote to bring light to the deepest, darkest struggles of millions of survivors and their families. I wrote because I refused to live a lie, to let a secret determine my destiny. I refused to keep quiet for the good of the family. I wrote not only to help others heal, but to reclaim my power and voice. And if that makes some relatives embarrassed or uncomfortable or feel that I'm being selfish, I concluded, that is their problem.

For Gail, who was abused by her stepfather and her uncle, the road to resolution took ten years, a failed marriage, a new sense of independence, and a courageous leap of faith.

"I relived the abuse every day of my life for more than twenty years," she says. "I accepted less for myself in everything from the least delectable piece of food on the buffet to the least desirable man for my husband. That would reflect how I felt about myself and what I felt I deserved." Today she sees herself and her world without the lens of anger or hatred or loathing that had colored her view for so long. "These days I feel strong, and I like my reflection in the mirror. I do not attribute every mistake or behavior to the abuse."

Gail did eventually tell her mother about her uncle's abuse. And at sixteen, in a fit of anger, she confronted and even came to blows with her stepfather. In college, she would candidly tell potential boyfriends, "There's something you ought to know before you love me. . . ."

From her actions, you would think that Gail had resolved the issues surrounding her past. But when she was twenty-seven and her first child was born, depression gripped her quickly and tightly. Then came thoughts of killing herself. She felt that God must have hated her and that her child would be better off without "a depressed and shameful mother." What saved her? Protecting her baby, and the thought that hell might be even worse than life on earth. Knowing that she was deeply troubled, Gail sought counseling on her own. The journal entry at the start of this chapter came five years after she checked herself into a mental health center for a month and began her work toward resolution.

ROADS TO RESOLUTION

Resolution can mean different things for different people. It can mean pressing charges or filing a civil suit. It can mean confronting or reconciling with an abuser and others who were aware of the abuse but did nothing to help. It can mean cutting ties to dysfunctional family members or situations and developing new, healthy relationships. It can mean forgiving and it can mean letting go.

For Gail, and for so many of the survivors I interviewed, resolution did not necessarily come from confrontation, nor, as we saw with Karla in

Chapter 7, did it come from the arrest and imprisonment of an abuser. Maya, whom we met in Chapter 3, found resolution not from an apology from her grandfather, who abused her, but from her parents' acknowledgment that the abuse actually happened. Tracey, from Chapter 4, found resolution through dance. Darlene, from Chapter 1, found it through her determination to keep children safe.

There is no one-size-fits-all approach to turning this corner. There are too many stages of denial, anger, healing, and pain. Mental health experts and survivor advocates recognize that the steps toward resolving a history of abuse are just as unique as a therapeutic treatment plan. And they are careful to let survivors determine that plan.

You are not likely to find, for example, a therapist pushing a client to confront an abuser, disclose abuse to family members, or forgive. For some survivors, the pressure to do so can be traumatizing in itself. "I ask people what they want to get out of therapy," says Maelinda Turner, the social worker, "and then I help them find it." If your therapist tries to convince you that you have only one route to resolving the many complicated, personal, and painful issues that are unique to you, find another therapist.

But while there is no one solution, there are a few paths that I heard survivors, therapists, and spiritual healers mention again and again:

* Confrontation
* Accountability and amends
* Faith and forgiveness

I explore these options in the following sections.

CONFRONTATION

Confrontation is letting the abuser know that you know what he or she did to you, and that it was illegal and morally wrong. That you did not deserve to be abused, and that it was not your fault. It is explaining how the abuser's actions affected your life. And it is telling how those actions made you feel. You can also tell the abuser how you want him or her to be accountable for these actions: acknowledgment, an apology, or a way to make amends (see the section below). You can give that person an opportunity to respond, but understand that he or she may not, or that the response may not be one you want to hear. Once you've said your piece, don't feel obligated to stick around.

Mental health professionals stress that, unlike telling someone about your abuse, confrontation is not a prerequisite to healing. While it can be a useful tool, confrontation will not affect a sexual abuser's mental disorder, nor will it change his behavior. As I explained in Chapter 7, "Challenging Abusers," behavioral changes can happen only if the abuser is in treatment and under supervision.

While confrontation is something you do for your own benefit, it is important that you understand the benefit you are seeking. You should never feel pressured to confront the person who abused you. It is a decision you must make on your own after much reflection, and it must be a decision you are comfortable with.

If you do want to confront your abuser, do so with the guidance of a professional. Don't worry if it has been years since the abuse took place. As Rhea Almeida of the Institute for Family Services says, "Some victims take a long time to begin to get the idea that they can challenge oppression." And don't stress yourself out trying to predict what might happen if you do. The book *The Courage to Heal*, which has an excellent section on this subject, "Disclosures and Confrontations," suggests that the aftermath can span a range of possibilities:

> *Women fear that a disclosure will cause a cataclysm: their mother will go insane, their father will kill himself, their aunt will divorce their uncle, the principal will fire the teacher. And sometimes such extreme reactions or major upheavals do happen. But it is also possible that very little will change. Whole families may pretend nothing was ever said.* [1]

You can find some questions to guide you in confronting an abuser in the "Help Yourself" section at the end of this chapter.

Your therapist can help mediate a confrontation. Almeida explained that when one client's mother suggested that she see her ailing father before he died, the client said she would do so only if the father went into treatment. Both parents ended up attending some of the client's group sessions, where the client read her letter confronting them before the entire group. "She said it was the most healing experience she'd ever had," Almeida says. Not every confrontation goes so smoothly, as Tracey's experience, below, shows.

A Rocky, but Useful, Confrontation

Tracey, the sister we met in Chapter 4 who found healing through dance, had tolerated her father's abuse for ten years, until at nineteen she resisted and he stopped. "He started by having me kiss him on the mouth, then with the tongue," says Tracey, who is now thirty-one. "That progressed to fondling and sucking my breasts. He explained that in different cultures, fathers did it with their daughters to prepare them" for sex. Her father also victimized her emotionally. "One day he told me that he had taken his gun to his job and he was going to kill his boss and kill himself but then he thought of me and didn't. He said I was the only person in the house who understood him."

Tracey kept the abuse to herself. In college, after seeing several therapists, she began to study dance as a therapeutic art form. She is now working on her doctorate in dance. She had never thought to disclose the abuse to her sister, Marilyn, who is older by two years and far more vocal. But one day, empowered by her dance and by years of therapy, Tracey told her story. Marilyn responded that their father had once tried to fondle her breasts, under the guise of checking for lumps. Marilyn said she became loud and hostile, and he backed off. Not long after that attempt, the sisters figured, is when he moved on to Tracey.

That revelation sent Tracey reeling. "It was as if I had had a personality more like hers, this wouldn't have happened so long," she says. "Like it was my fault. It depressed me to know that she had more power to make it stop and I didn't."

Tracey was convinced that her mother knew what had happened, and she and Marilyn decided to confront their parents. Marilyn fired off letters, "cursing them out and being really angry," Tracey says. That wasn't her style. Then the sisters arranged for their father to meet with them. Over dinner they told him that they knew about the abuse and that what he had done was wrong. His response? Tracey says, "Basically he said we should be lucky that he didn't kill us. He thought we should be happy. He said, 'I've heard about when women get raped. Well, you're alive.'" The sisters were appalled, but they pressed on.

When Marilyn suggested that the whole family should go into therapy, their father was quick to show remorse. "He said, 'You know, if you want me to say I'm sorry, I'm sorry.' I knew he didn't mean it. And then he said something like, 'The White man is not going to judge me. God is my only judge.'"

As disturbing as his response was, Tracey began to see that regardless of what he said, the experience was a form of closure. She moved on to her mother, who initially invoked religion: "She explained that this was the work of the devil, trying to get her to divorce my father, but she doesn't believe in divorce," Tracey says. About a year or so later, Tracey tried again.

She started by telling her mother how angry she was that the older woman was in denial. "She seemed shocked," Tracey says. "And then she said, 'Well, I did think—sometimes you would be watching television with your father and he would have his arm around you, and you were scrunching, like you just didn't look comfortable.'" Tracey asked her: "Mommy, why didn't you follow that gut feeling? Why didn't you ask or say something when you saw that?"

Her mother's response: She didn't want her husband to think she was jealous of her daughter. That was the final indignity for Tracey. She rarely sees her parents now.

As often happens, Tracey's confrontations did not lead either parent to accept responsibility for the abuse. But she still found the process useful. "It was helpful for me to get some insight on where they were coming from. And it made me start saying, 'I have to speak. I have to talk about this.' Because they are so in denial. Dance has been my weapon, or my voice."

ACCOUNTABILITY

Rhea Almeida recognizes that many survivors may face family denial, as Tracey did. That's why, in her New Jersey therapy center, you will often find survivors of sexual and domestic violence challenging and confronting abusers who are ordered by the courts to participate in group therapy. "This gives a person a chance to hear the community challenge an oppressor, even if it is not her oppressor," Almeida says. The goal is for survivors to see abusers held accountable for their actions.

The power in providing this substitute family dynamic is that it can help survivors resolve issues that their own families will not. "It's one thing for those who've been injured to learn to validate their feelings, to get out of depression," says Almeida, "but if there's never a conversation in the family about the fact that this guy was abusive, it is always an open wound. If the community or the church continues to elevate this guy with no discussion about what he's done, it creates a cutoff between the woman and her family and community. She has already healed but is being re-scarred by the fact that her community is in denial."

If abusers do acknowledge their offenses, Almeida encourages her clients to hold them accountable, too, "noting that an apology is simply not enough."

Borrowing from the concept behind South Africa's Truth and Reconciliation Commission, Almeida provides a forum, a group counseling session, in which the abuser reads a "letter of accountability" recalling each incident of abuse. Letters are crafted over months with the help of sponsors, or former group members, who help guide the abusers. "They might start out sketchy with one or two incidents, but the sponsor will ask questions and send them back again and again," Almeida says. The goal is for the abuser to come to see the pattern of abuse and its impact, listing dates, times, episodes of violation, abuses of power, and reactions. This approach is much like that of experts who work solely with abusers, except it is for the benefit of the survivor.

With accountability comes amends or reparations. Almeida has seen former abusers pay for her clients' therapy, college or graduate school, lost wages, and even school for the children of a client. "The thinking is, if you disrupt a life, you have to make up for a life," she says. Abusers have also donated money to rape and sexual abuse crisis centers. Noting that not everybody can afford to pay damages, Almeida suggests these other ways to make amends:

- Seek treatment
- Write an "accountability" letter and read it before the family (this should be done with the guidance of a counselor)
- Donate time and services to a community activism group
- Testify before the legislature for stronger statutes for abuse survivors
- Testify before the legislature to increase sexual abuse prevention programs in schools and for adults

FAITH AND FORGIVENESS

Nearly every survivor I interviewed spoke of faith and a need to forgive. As I sought healing through therapy, I struggled with the notion of forgiveness. I remember thinking, "How can I forgive a person who won't even acknowledge his offense, much less ask for forgiveness?" I was angered by the thought that here I was, the person offended, and I was obligated to do the work! In interviewing survivors, I found that I was not alone. Gail, for example, was torn and confused by the mixed messages she got about faith and church and from the adults around her.

"My mother made sure we were in church every Sunday," Gail says. "We sang in the choir and went to Bible school each week. My church wasn't a teaching church, it was a preaching church. And so the preacher was not somebody that you went to with your problems because he would talk about them in the next service. Then my uncle—the one who had abused me— ended up being my Bible School teacher, and I had to deal with the whole hypocrisy of that situation."

We African Americans are deeply spiritual people; our faith has helped so many of us survive the horrors of slavery and oppression. For many of us, faith is a cornerstone of our healing. Nearly every person I interviewed talked of a sustaining belief in a divine power. That's not surprising. The majority of Americans say they believe that a patient's religious faith can have a positive effect on his or her recovery from an illness or injury.[2] But as a survivor of sexual abuse, a trauma of the mind, body, and spirit, I found that my faith was tested. I know that forgiveness is a powerful force toward resolution. But it has taken time to embrace this concept and to actually practice it.

First I needed to understand what it means to forgive. I started with the dictionary. *Webster's Collegiate,* Tenth Edition, defines it as "to give up resentment of or claim to requital for," "to grant relief from payment of," and "to cease to feel resentment against." Simple enough. But what about forgiveness within the context of faith? What about that sense of Christian obligation that annoyed me? I understood why Rhea Almeida and many therapists avoid emphasizing forgiveness. "It is far more empowering to focus on accountability," Almeida says. In fact, when a client tells her that she's being pressured by her church to forgive, Almeida suggests that she find another church. For a better understanding of forgiveness, I sought guidance from three divinely gifted healers whose approaches to spirituality I respect enormously: Marcia Dyson, the noted minister, scholar, and social critic who in her writings has challenged our churches to be more receptive and responsive to women; Carmen Murray, a Detroit Public Schools social worker who is also a licensed minister for prayer and missions at Detroit's Mt. Zion Church; and San Francisco social worker Maelinda Turner, who holds a degree in divinity and practices metaphysical healing techniques like Reiki.

Each shared her perspective, clarifying the notion of forgiveness and shattering some misconceptions about what it means to forgive. Their guidance stems from Christian principles rooted in their belief in God and their interpretation of the Bible. But the lessons they share are universal. Here are some of the highlights from our talks.

Marcia Dyson acknowledges that our religious institutions often expect women to forgive the infractions against them but do not expect the same from men if they are violated. "If men were sexually assaulted at the rate, at gunpoint, with hands at throat, the way women were and are, the laws would be changed and forgiveness would not be the first thing upon their lips," she says. "But when it's the bodies of women, we are told to have conversation, consideration, compassion, contemplation." She suggests that churches set up ministries and healing circles to deal with sexual abuse, and that survivors focus on forgiving themselves first.

- **It's not about the offender.** "Forgiveness is not to release the person who did harm but to release the person who has been harmed. So often it is not that we cannot forgive a perpetrator but we cannot forgive ourselves. We tell ourselves that we put ourselves in a position to receive the assault: if you hadn't acted that way, dressed that way, been at the wrong place, kept quiet about it. Knowing that *it wasn't your fault* is part of forgiving yourself."

- **Take your time.** "It's possible for someone to forgive a perpetrator immediately, based on their relationship with God and the maturity of their spirituality. I'm not there. Even as a minister, I cannot readily say that if it happened to me or my daughter that my immediate response would be compassion. My first reaction is that this man be castrated first and then go to trial. I suggest time as a part of the ritual of healing."

- **You don't need to be asked.** "Regardless of whether a person confesses, it doesn't change the reality for the person who was offended. To expect somebody to confess when they don't even understand that they've got a pathology is ludicrous. You cannot place responsibility for your peace of mind—your soul's salvation—upon their response."

- **To forgive does not mean to forget.** "We wouldn't want to forget. That means we would not be advocates; we would not be lobbyists for more stringent laws to stop this from happening. We wouldn't have international coalitions to help women who are violated."

- **Churches can show the way.** "Every church should have a sister minister—not assistant minister that acknowledges the anniversaries or fries the chicken or teaches Sunday school, but a minister who administers the rituals of healing: confession, forgiveness, laying on of hands. Churches should allow a person to confess—to acknowledge that this thing happened. And when we acknowledge it, hopefully we are in a circle where we have some healers, those who can lay human hands on you. You also need to be able to confess your sins and errors, knowing that God is faithful and just and can forgive your sins. By sin, I'm talking not about the sin of having been assaulted, but the sin of feeling like you are the reason this happened to you. The sin of allowing anything in your life to disconnect you from God. "

Maelinda Turner's clients bring a range of spiritual beliefs to her, from the metaphysical to the traditional. What's common, though, is how much her clients, most of whom are African American, depend on prayer. Turner helps abuse survivors recognize that they already have what they need to help themselves. "People who have survived this trauma have an innate strength and ability to heal. My job is to help them see it."

- **Don't underestimate the power of faith.** "It is your faith and spirituality that got you through the situation in the first place. For many people, faith and healing are inseparable. The role of faith in healing itself is such an intangible thing. You can't measure it. You can't even define it. But you can recognize that there is something bigger in this world, and that you're a part of it."

- **Don't force the issue.** "Nobody can force forgiveness—whether a therapist or the church. It happens naturally. Remember that the ultimate goal is to move on and not wallow in the past. The experience will always be a part of you but doesn't have to control your life."

- **Go easy on yourself.** "Sisters who beat themselves up for not being able to forgive should know that it is another form of abuse and self-hate. You feel you're not worthy. Not Christian. Sex abuse already teaches you shame and self-hatred. You can't try to heal and beat up on yourself. That's taking on the abuser's role."

- **Stay true and loyal to yourself.** "One of the lessons of sex abuse is not to abandon yourself like other people have. Somewhere along the way many survivors felt abandoned because somebody didn't take care of them. The healing process is about a commitment to taking care of yourself for the rest of your life."

Carmen Murray says that forgiveness is a matter of will. "Many times people think forgiveness is about feeling. But you will never feel like forgiving somebody who has victimized you."

- **Forgiveness is an act of faith.** "It is faith in a God that would allow abuse to happen, and faith that God would deal with the victimizer and heal the abused."

- **Forgiveness brings freedom.** "Forgiveness means to release or set free. Intellectually you can confront, sit the person down, write letters, but if you are not going through the pain and release of forgiveness you are not free. Even if the person dies, you are not free. Forgiveness brings freedom to trust, freedom from fear and suspicion, freedom from bitterness, freedom from guilt and shame, freedom from embarrassment, freedom to tell the truth. Forgiveness is like turning the light on the secrecy of abuse."

- **Forgiveness is empowering.** "It is a powerful thing to be able to say, 'I choose to forgive.' You didn't have a choice in being victimized. Here you have a choice."

- **Leave the vengeance to God.** "Oftentimes we want to determine how God deals with perpetrators. We want to set the sentence and the punishment. Some will deal with the court system, of course, but for so many others, if the person who has victimized you never has an understanding of the depth of your hurt, they cannot pay. Even if you blow their head off, you're not making them pay. Know that God handles this. That's where faith comes in."

These are the kinds of words that survivors need to hear in their churches, temples, and mosques. So many survivors are in deep, deep pain and have estranged themselves from religious institutions because they cannot find the support and welcome embrace of spiritual leaders and ministers that says, "I understand." All too often, our female-supported, male-dominated places of worship ignore or dismiss instances when women or children are victimized by the men in their communities. In fact, as the Catholic Church crisis has shown, churches, often shielded by silence and secrecy, can be where abuse thrives. Dyson reminds us that we need to change the balance of power in our churches: "While male ministers give plenty of lip service to the church's reliance on Black women, that recognition does not spur them to envision a church where justice for women prevails."[3] Our places of worship need to encourage discussion about sexual violence in general, about race, power, and oppression, and about respecting the rights of women and children. Leaders need to report suspicions or disclosures of abuse so that those involved can get the appropriate help. In addition to the ministries that Dyson suggested, all spiritual leaders should receive special training in counseling. There is enormous untapped potential to address sexual abuse in the sacred places to which many of us turn in our times of greatest need.

COMING TO TERMS WITH ABUSERS

You may determine that you don't want to press charges, file a civil suit, or confront or even forgive a childhood sexual abuser. It's your call. What's most important is that your decision is based not on fear or shame, but on what's most comfortable for you.

What's left? Coming to terms with abusers. Whether you confront or not, there is a need to acknowledge what the person did and how it affected you. Even if you write it in a letter and mail it. Or write it down and burn it up. Even using a therapist or a trusted friend as a stand-in helps. Meditations, affirmations—whatever works. It is most important that you have the chance to place the blame for what happened on the person who caused it, and to articulate the damage that person caused.

How long does it take to resolve these issues? "It takes as long as it takes," Rhea Almeida says. She knows a client is making progress when the balance between the trauma and the resilience shifts so that the trauma becomes less and less and the resilience becomes greater, she says. "I don't want people to be dead to the trauma in their lives, but I want them to be able to move beyond it and externalize it and take charge of it." She helps clients see that they are already in conflict with their families, even if the issue of abuse has not been raised. Davis sees progress when a client can bring the abuse into the open and stand up to hostile family members. "You can say, 'I know I'm aggravating and I won't let this rest, but this is me and you've got to accept me for what I am,'" she says.

Gail's journey to resolution takes her through many of the issues that we have explored. Hers is a torturous trip filled with the pain of abuse, the loss of family ties, and the confusion and self-doubt that many survivors know well. But at nearly every step we see a resilient sister emerging, fighting her way through the betrayals and contradictions and loneliness to find peace with her past and her God and a measure of happiness in her life. Gail, soft-spoken with a sharp mind and dry wit, courageously agreed to let us follow her soul-searching and progress through some very candid entries in her journals. Before she shared her journals with me, she says, she took some time to flip through them and saw her remarkable progress. "I can't believe that person was me."

GAIL'S STORY: "DEAR GOD, PLEASE SHOW ME THE WAY"

At twenty-seven, for the first time in her life, Gail sought counseling. Her therapist recommended a residential treatment center. There she was diagnosed as clinically depressed and a doctor prescribed Prozac. Giving birth to her daughter had sent Gail into depression, but also had given her the will to survive. "I believed that mothers screwed up the lives of their children and I did not want to hurt my child. But then I thought, 'Who will protect her from people like my stepfather and uncle?'"

2/8/91
Well, I did it finally. I have checked into a mental health facility. I hope I can get past this depression and shame and guilt. . . . I did it for the baby as well as myself. . . . I know all too well how parents can hurt and harm their children even when they think they're doing things in their children's best interest. Coming here was the second hardest thing I've ever had to do. The first was writing Mom that letter telling her what _____ did to me, even if I didn't tell her everything. I think for the first time that Mom realized just how intense my depression is. She always said I could handle anything. This time she was wrong.

In many ways, Gail held her mother responsible for much of her pain and feared that she would be like her. When Gail was fourteen, she described in a letter how her stepfather "would sneak into my room at night when I was sleeping and put his fingers in me." After reading Gail's letter, Gail's mother told her she would "handle it," but Gail's stepfather, who had moved out, stayed away for only a week. When he returned, letting himself in with his own key, he continued the abuse. Gail was left to fend for herself. "When I protested, he would tell me that no one would believe me and that my mom would not love me anymore." For years, she believed him.

2/25/91

Today I told my darkest secrets. I guess that means I'm getting better. Doc says that conflict within me about feeling responsible for what _____ and _____ did is not my fault. Children can't be responsible for making adult decisions. . . . Even though my body reacted in the way it's supposed to when touched it doesn't mean that I liked what happened or that I wanted it to happen. If I did like the sexual pleasure it brought it was not my fault because I was the child. . . . I can't release myself from the guilt because I knew it was wrong. I sought sex from cousins and I knew which ones would be safe and which wouldn't. I continue to pay for my sins each time I have sex with my husband. Mom told me that an uncle had touched her. I asked because her behavior matched the classic behavior described in the book I'm reading. I'm surprised she didn't try to hide it. And that she told me he used his finger. That's terrible but at least I know that Mom understands the guilt and self-hate that stems from it. I love my mom and I understand now why she couldn't bring herself to talk to me about the incest. She was denying it all. All these years I thought she didn't believe me. Or that she loved _____ more. Now I understand. . . . When my baby grows up I want her to know about incest so if anyone tries anything she will know about it and come to me with it right away.

While in therapy, Gail learned that many of the behaviors she exhibited stemmed from her abuse: the many sexual partners, self-mutilation, smoking, and drinking herself into blackouts. When she asked her mother whether she also had been abused, her mother confirmed Gail's suspicion, "blurting it out like it had been building up all her life." That was the first and the last that her mother spoke about her own experience. "I now understand my mother's limitation and why she was so unhappy," Gail says. "I understand why we went through a period when we weren't friends at all. I know she did the best she could. If she had not been abused herself, she might have kept him away."

8/17/91

Tarik [Gail's husband] *and I have been arguing about his wanting to go out with other women. . . . He believes there is nothing wrong with it as long as he doesn't have sex. I disagree. . . . He admitted that while I was away he wanted to kill himself and the baby. He felt I wasn't there for him and that he needed to find another female companion. I find it hard to believe that a man who desires other women and wants permission from his wife to go out with them, does not have a particular woman in mind. . . . I left. . . . Put the baby in the car and drove and refused to speak with him for two days. . . . He seemed content to begin preparing a life alone or at least without me. He said our marriage was stale. . . . This past week I went to see him and he just wanted sex. . . . My marriage has lost its most important ingredient—trust.*

Once Tarik asked Gail just how many sexual partners she had had. They counted together, and the number approached one hundred. Most of these were while she was drunk or high. "I had always felt like that little girl was now the one in power," she says. "I had the power of deciding when I wanted sex and I could get it from any man."

When they were dating, Gail had told Tarik about the abuse. She told him about how her stepfather would come into the house and watch her sleep. She told him how she would be awakened at night by his hands under the blanket. "I used to tuck in the covers tightly before going to bed so he couldn't get to me," she remembers. She told him about how she was made to babysit her cousins even though her uncle was home, and how, when the cousins would take a nap, he would "climb on top of me and put his penis in me and take it out before he came in his hands." Gail says she shared her past with Tarik "because I felt like a damaged piece of goods, and he needed to know the damage." After they were married, Gail began to have flashbacks, often when she and Tarik were having sex. Tarik encouraged her to drink beforehand. "He said it was better when I was intoxicated," Gail says. When she returned from the treatment center, he encouraged her to skip the Prozac, which diminishes sex drive. She tried to accommodate him (they had a second child), but eventually she realized that he was doing nothing to accommodate her. Soon he began to stay out late and come home drunk. "I felt betrayed, disappointed, and abandoned," Gail says. "I felt he was weak, like my uncle and stepfather."

4/5/94

He's gone away from my heart. My problems have overshadowed our love. This I cannot blame him for—no man can live with incest or its victim. I can't live with it, either. I've been slowly dying for years. . . . Condemned to die a shameful death not unlike the life I've lived. God I won't be seeing. . . . Like everyone I've loved, mostly my children, I've let down, unable to live beyond my past. . . . My only good is my children. I love them enough to let them go. . . . Let hell have me in death as in life. . . . No father, no husband, no children and no life.

4/8/94

It's a good thing I wrote my feelings down. On paper I can see the stupidity in ending one's life. From this day forward I will accept and cherish life with all of its good as well as its bad. There is no more room for Tarik in my life . . . he hasn't been there for me in a long time. I haven't been there for me. Now this has changed. I celebrate my children and I welcome change. . . . I give myself to God. I open my heart.

After several fits and starts, Gail left Tarik for the last time. She took her girls and moved in with her sister. She found her own place, a car, and a job, things she would have never done when she was with her husband. "I gave too much of myself to him and gave up too many dreams trying to hold on to my marriage," she says, "when there was nothing I could have done to prevent it from falling apart."

5/30/94

My fears: I fear I haven't the faith to do as I see; I fear to give my life to God. Why? My faith is weak. What must I do then? Pray, and read my Bible. . . . Dear God, please show me the way.

Gail's family was deeply religious, and for years she had convinced herself that it was she, not her abusers, who were wrong. "I once wrote a letter to God with a bunch of questions," she says. "'Why did this happen to me? Was I evil?' I learned from church about some people going to heaven and some going to hell. For the longest time, I had thought that I was in the bunch of folks that was going to hell."

After she and her husband divorced, Gail tried teaching and later joined the sexual assault crisis center where she now works. She lives with her two girls now, single and at peace with herself, with her God and with her family. "Today I tolerate my uncle, but I don't hang around him," she says. "I decided a long time ago that my aunt was important and that I did not want to hurt her. I have the feeling of empowerment. I am not afraid of him. I see his feeble weakness, but I no longer hate him. I have stayed away from my stepfather. He doesn't come around anymore—he's very sick—but when he used to, my children and I would simply leave."

She remembers how much the abuse once consumed her. "I used to dream of how I would kill him," she says of her stepfather. "The anger and hate made my life miserable. I remember clearly the day I drop-kicked him in the balls as hard as I could, and when he went down, I punched him in the mouth. That felt so good. But I had to decide to let go of the hate because I realized that I couldn't love anybody. I needed to forgive because the abuse happened a long time ago, but I was still living it every day."

Gail has forgiven herself, she says, and has never been more hopeful that she and her family can find resolution. "I do not sit and dwell on it. Being an active participant in the movement to end sexual violence channels my passion to hold perpetrators accountable. I have two daughters in the highest-risk age category for child sex abuse. I've been open about the work that I do. They've spent time in the office volunteering. They know how strongly I feel about protecting them from sexual violence. I see happy children develop as I would have had I not been abused, and it's a blessing. I confronted both my abusers. My uncle denied he had ever had intercourse with me, and my stepfather's response was to offer me anything I wanted if I'd let him have sex with me. This helped me understand how sick he really is. About a year ago, my sister, mother, and I ended up talking about my stepfather and how uncomfortable they were allowing children around him. I shared with them for the first time my confrontation and what he told me. I guess as a family we will continue to heal together. There are still more secrets we have yet to discuss."

Perhaps through Gail, her family will indeed come together to heal. But it's clear that whether or not they choose to join her, this is a journey Gail is prepared to make on her own.

LETTING GO, LETTING GOD

I see myself in many of the survivors I have interviewed. Perhaps you do, too. Like Gail, Shantel, Darlene, and Maya, like Robert and Carol, I am among the healers—those who work to raise awareness and help others recover from child sexual abuse. Looking back on my journey—from the day I cried in that sister circle six years ago to the day that I ended therapy last year—I had no light-bulb moment in which all the pain went away, but the more I understood the toll of sexual abuse on our families, and sexual abuse in my family, the more I accepted and appreciated myself and others—imperfections and all.

I now know that I have nothing to prove because that little girl was groped in a closet so many years ago. After all, she was one smart cookie for getting me as far as she did. I told her that she done good, and she went away quite pleased with herself, for a change. She left it to me to accept my past, to ask for help, do the hard work to heal. To share with my husband so he could understand. To ensure that my son knows that he is our priority, and that he has rights—even as a child.

It was not easy to get here. And even now, I know I still have work to do.

But I start each day seeking joy. And if the past gets in the way, I merely look to it for the lessons it brings, and then I move on. That's what I've learned from healing work, and from the courageous survivors I spoke with. That's what I've tried to share.

When we value our children, respect our worth as women, stand up to our men, and know our legacy, we can look beyond our fears and accept our responsibility to keep one another safe. Our future depends on it—the sanity and survival of us all.

Before I began writing this book, I would often think about confronting my uncle for abusing me. I was angry that he did not acknowledge and take responsibility for his actions. I was angry that my family was not outraged by what he had done. I was angry because of the work I had to do to untangle the effects of abuse from my life.

But then my mother reminded me how, when I disclosed to her and she went to confront him, my biggest fear was that others in the family would know. I was so embarrassed that I desperately wanted to keep it a secret. I realized then that resolution for me would be not in confrontation, but in understanding the silence surrounding the crime of sexual abuse, especially within our families.

One day I asked myself, "What would happen if I just stopped wasting my time and energy on anger and turned it to something else?" I immediately sensed a load lifting from my shoulders, so I decided to let it all go. That simple act made room for me to begin researching and writing this book.

As part of my therapy several years ago, I wrote an enraged, teary letter to my uncle. *"I hate you!"* it started. It went on to describe how he had hurt me and how saddened I was that he denied what he did. That was my first step toward resolution.

Over the next few years, as I continued healing work and began to research and write about sexual abuse, I wrote three more letters to him, to help me understand and express long-unspoken feelings. After I finished each letter, I would tuck it away.

About a year ago, as I prepared to write this book, I found all the letters and read them together for the first time. I was immediately struck by not only my personal growth but also my ability to step back and see the issue of sexual abuse not just in terms of my own experience, but in the larger context of a vicious cycle of epidemic proportions.

My first letter portrayed the little girl who was hurt and confused. By the second letter, I was more angry than sad. By the third, I'd started research for the book, and I had begun to learn about not just survivors, but also sexual abusers. I understood that child sexual abuse often stems from a mental disorder—an inability to control the impulse to victimize children. But I also began to hold him accountable

I wrote the fourth letter as I began to write the book. It reflects a much deeper perspective on the issue of sexual abuse and its impact on survivors and families. The anger is gone, replaced by insight and compassion and a demand for accountability. The empowered, informed adult survivor who wrote the fourth letter is light-years from the hurt little girl who wrote the first.

At one point I planned to send my uncle all four letters, then I decided not to send any. Instead, I thought, I'll send this book to him, and to others in my family. It is never too late to begin healing.

HELP YOURSELF

─────────────────────────────────

Accountability and Responsibility

Confronting an Abuser It is important to know that this experience is for nobody else but you. It's also important to know why you want to confront the abuser and perhaps others who knew about the abuse but did not come to your aid. According to mental health experts, the book *The Courage to Heal,* and VOICES in Action, Inc., here are some issues to consider in confronting:[4]

- **Purpose.** What do you want to get out of this experience? Think about what you hope to accomplish and how your actions—regardless of the response of the abuser—will help you move on with your life. Use your stated purpose as a beacon to guide you through this process.

- **Method.** Confrontation does not have to happen in person. Survivors have confronted in person, by phone, by letter, and by e-mail—even by telegram. Choose the method you feel most comfortable using.

- **Message.** What will you say? Write it down. List points you want to cover, in order of importance. Have the list with you when you confront.

- **Location.** If you want a face-to-face meeting, find a neutral spot: a public place such as a park, or the home of a supportive relative or friend. You can even meet in your therapist's office. Don't go to the home of the abuser, and don't meet in your home.

- **Reaction.** Think about the tricks, tactics, or comments the abuser might use to catch you off guard. Think about how your action might affect your relationship with the rest of your family.

- **Extra support.** Consider having a friend or relative with you. If your confrontation is face-to-face, your friend can be far enough away to see but not hear your discussion.

- **Safety.** If the abuser has a history of physical violence, it may not be safe to confront.

- **Your expectations.** Don't expect the abuser to suddenly acknowledge or apologize. In fact, he or she may become very angry or call you a liar. Think about the worst thing that might happen, and prepare for that.

- **Your response.** What will you say if the abuser denies it? If the abuser blames you? If the abuser becomes angry? What if the person apologizes? Think about what you might do in several circumstances.

- **An exit plan.** Think about how you would like the meeting or conversation to end, and how you would end it if you became uncomfortable. Consider saying something like, "If you don't stop talking to me like this, I am going to leave."

- **Timing.** Know that you can decide to abort your plans to confront at any time.

- **Afterward.** What will you do when it's over? Plan to have the rest of your day free. Have someone with you for support.

It is even possible to confront the deceased. Many mental health professionals suggest writing letters or role-playing the confrontation with a counselor or a supporter. Some survivors have even visited gravesites, and others have made tape recordings or videos. These exercises can even be useful for those who, for whatever reason, do not want to interact with the abuser but want to speak their piece. If you take this approach, still make sure to consider Purpose, Method, Message, and Afterward from the list above.

A Letter of Loss One of the most painful losses that stems from sexual abuse is the ability to have intimacy. Carol, who is thirty-six (Chapter 5), has never had a boyfriend. Never been in love. Never made love. "Not that those things define me," she says, "but they are a part of maturity, womanhood, and adulthood. I have a real fear of getting too physical or intimate with a guy, only to open my eyes and see my father."

With her psychological insight and spiritual awakening, Carol sought to understand her father. "As part of the process of healing and forgiveness, I've had to separate the man—my father—from the sin—childhood sexual abuse," she says, without minimizing her own experience. "Yes, the acts of sexual abuse are heinous, but I've had to wonder what type of life experiences would compel a man, a father, to initiate sexual contact with his daughter. I believe there are demons that still haunt him from his childhood, and that my father carries a tremendous amount of guilt and shame." It is that perspective, she says, that has allowed her to move on with her life.

Even though Carol cut ties with her family after her mother suggested she "let it go," Carol felt compelled to write to her father about all that she had lost because of his abuse. She mailed it to him on June 3, 2001. In it, she listed these losses:

- *Innocence.*
- *Ability to trust (I'm always on guard against anyone who could hurt me or take something precious from me).*
- *Ability to experience emotional and sexual maturity as a normal progression from childhood to adolescence to adulthood.*
- *Chances for an open, trustworthy relationship with you and others.*
- *Respect for you and others.*
- *Desire to be influenced by family members or others.*
- *Desire or openness to share problems, issues, or intimate details of my life and longings.*
- *Ability to trust my own instincts (is what I'm feeling really real?).*
- *Ability or freedom to feel emotions.*
- *I had lost a loving and protective image of God.*
- *I've lost the ability to trust and feel safe when entering intimate relationships with men. (For that matter, I've never experienced true intimacy with another man! Hell, I'm thirty-five! Do you have any idea what kinda mind trips that takes me on?!)*
- *I've lost a desire to have children.*
- *I've lost thirty-five years' worth of opportunities to have a loving and enlightening mother-daughter relationship; I've had to seek nurturance*

*and encouragement in the arms, eyes, and words of other women who are
not my mother.*

Her father has yet to respond.

Drafting a Family Code of Conduct   Earlier in this book, I referred to an
unspoken family trust that our kin are a source of nurturing, sharing, and
safety. But not everybody knows that being family comes with these basic
rights. And when some don't honor the rights, not everybody knows what
to do. So just what are the ground rules for belonging to a family? In her
therapy sessions, Janet Davis, the Harlem social worker, helps families clar-
ify their obligations, often to restore the trust that has been broken because
of abuse and years of silence. "Sometimes you have to spell it out," Davis
says. "You can say, 'We need to love each other,' but some folks don't really
know what that means. It helps to have it listed so that people can make a
commitment to upholding the family responsibilities." If we were to make a
list of those responsibilities, what would be on it?

On the following page is an example of a Family Code of Conduct,
which is based on Davis's suggestions. Use it as a guide to draft your own
code, adding other obligations based on your family's needs. Enlist other relatives to help shape the list, and encourage discussion about why each item
belongs. You can have a spiritual leader or a respected elder facilitate the dialogue. After discussion, have each member sign the code as an indication of
support for family unity and strength. Call a family meeting, or use your
next family gathering or reunion as an opportunity to commit or reaffirm
what you deserve and are entitled to from one another.

The _____ Family
Code of Conduct

1. To keep each family member safe
2. To communicate openly and honestly
3. To show compassion and be supportive when people need me
4. To treat others with respect
5. To respect the boundaries of others
6. To point out when others don't live up to this commitment
7. To speak up when somebody's actions are not appropriate

Signed:

_____   _____

_____   _____

_____   _____

_____   _____

_____

Date: _____

From *No Secrets, No Lies: How Black Families Can Heal from Sexual Abuse,* by Robin D. Stone © 2004.

RESOURCES

ADVOCACY / HELP FOR CHILDREN

To report child sexual abuse, call the police. Or look up your city or county division of child protective services or children's services (the name may be slightly different). Start with your telephone directory. In some areas you can be directed to local services by calling 311 or 211. If you can't find the appropriate agency, your state coalition against sexual assault (see below) or one of these national organizations can direct you.

ChildHelp USA—National Child Abuse Hotline
ChildHelp USA National Headquarters
15757 N. 78th Street
Scottsdale, AZ 85260
(408) 922-8212
(800) 4-A-Child; (800) 422-4453
www.childhelpusa.org

An organization that aims to meet the physical, emotional, educational, and spiritual needs of abused and neglected children. ChildHelp's Web site includes a state-by-state listing of phone numbers to report child sexual abuse.

National Children's Alliance
1612 K Street NW, Suite 500
Washington, DC 20006
(800) 239-9950
www.nca-online.org

A nonprofit organization that helps communities establish and improve children's advocacy centers, which serve abused children and their families.

Darkness to Light
247 Meeting Street
Charleston, SC 29401
(843) 965-5444
www.darkness2light.org

A nonprofit organization that seeks to reduce child sexual abuse nationally through education and public awareness aimed at adults. D2L's mission is to shift responsibility for preventing child sexual abuse from children to adults.

The National Children's Advocacy Center
210 Pratt Avenue
Huntsville, AL 35801
(256) 533-5437
www.nationalcac.org

A nonprofit agency providing prevention, intervention, and treatment services to physically and sexually abused children and their families.

National Center for Missing and Exploited Children
Charles B. Wang International Children's Building
699 Prince Street
Alexandria, VA 22314-3175
(703) 274-3900
(703) 274-2200
(800) THE-LOST; (800) 843-5678
www.missingkids.com

An organization that helps families and professionals prevent the abduction, endangerment, and sexual exploitation of children. Helps law enforcement in the prosecution of criminals who prey on children.

The Children's Defense Fund
25 E Street, NW
Washington, DC 20001
(202) 628-8787
www.childrensdefense.org
E-mail: cdfinfo@childrensdefense.org

A national organization that advocates for children in America, with particular attention to the needs of the poor, children of color, and children with disabilities.

ADVOCACY / HELP FOR SURVIVORS

Rape, Abuse & Incest National Network

635B Pennsylvania Avenue SE
Washington, DC 20003
(202) 544-1034, ext. 1
(800) 656-HOPE; (800) 656-4673
www.rainn.org

One of the nation's largest and most recognized anti-sexual-assault organizations, which carries out programs to prevent sexual assault, help victims, and ensure that rapists are brought to justice. Offers twenty-four-hour crisis intervention online and by phone. Can refer you to a nearby rape crisis center.

Voices in Action

P.O. Box 13
Newtonsville, OH 45158
(773) 327-1500
(800) 7-VOICE-8; (800) 786-4238
www.voices-action.org

An international organization that provides assistance to adult victims of child sexual abuse. Provides referrals to self-help groups, therapists, and other resources.

Survivors of Incest Anonymous

World Service Office, P.O. Box 190
Benson, MD 21018-9998
(410) 893-3322
www.siawso.org

An organization for men and women ages eighteen and older who were sexually abused as children.

Generation Five
2 Massasoit Street
San Francisco, CA 94110
(415) 285-6658
www.generationfive.org

An organization that works to halt and mend the intergenerational impact of child sexual abuse on children, families, and individuals through organizing and public action.

The Safer Society Foundation, Inc.
P.O. Box 340
Brandon, VT 05733
(802) 247-3132
Sexual Abuser Treatment Referral Line: (802) 247-3132
www.safersociety.org

A nonprofit national research advocacy and referral center. Offers a wide selection of books, cassettes, and videos for offenders, victims, family members, and clinicians, addressing the prevention and treatment of sexual abuse.

Black Women's Health Imperative
(formerly the National Black Women's Health Project)
(202) 548-4000
600 Pennsylvania Avenue SE, Suite 310
Washington, D.C. 20003
www.blackwomenshealth.org

The leading education, research, advocacy, and leadership development institution for Black women's health concerns.

National Organization for Women
202-331-9002
733 15th Street NW, 2nd floor
Washington, D.C. 20005
www.now.org

The nation's leading feminist organization, which advocates for equal rights and to end violence against women. Web site provides links to local chapters.

Men Can Stop Rape
P.O. Box 57144
Washington, DC 20037
(202) 265-6530
www.mencanstoprape.org

An organization that empowers male youth and the institutions that serve them to work as allies with women in preventing rape and other forms of men's violence.

Rosa Parks Sexual Assault Crisis Center
4182 S. Western Avenue
Los Angeles, CA 90062
(223) 290-4119

A center that provides counseling and support for children and adults.

VDay
http://www.vday.org

A global movement that promotes creative events to increase awareness, raise money, and revitalize the spirit of existing antiviolence organizations to stop sexual and domestic violence against women and girls.

National Center for Victims of Crime
2000 M Street NW, Suite 480
Washington, DC 20036
(202) 467-8700
(800) FYI-CALL; (800) 394-2255
www.ncvc.org

A leading resource and advocacy organization for crime victims. Works with grassroots organizations and criminal justice agencies to help victims rebuild their lives.

LEGAL HELP

For more information, see the HelpYourself section at the end of Chapter 7.

The National Crime Victim Bar Association
2000 M Street NW, Suite 480
Washington, DC 20036
(800) FYI-CALL
(202) 467-8753
www.victimbar.org
E-mail: victimbar@ncvc.org

A network of attorneys and other professionals that provides referrals to local attorneys in victim-related litigation. An affiliate of the National Center for Victims of Crime.

Justice for Children
733 15th Street NW, Suite 214
Washington, DC 20005
(202) 462-4688
www.jfcadvocacy.org

An organization that advocates for children's protection from abuse. Maintains a lawyers referral list by state.

The Martindale-Hubbell Lawyer Locator
www.martindale.com

The online version of the advertising directory for lawyers. Lets you search by geographical area, name, and specialty, among other options.

National Organization for Women Legal Defense and Education Fund
395 Hudson Street
NewYork, NY 10014
(212) 925-6635
www.nowldef.org

This organization, which is separate from NOW, provides a helpline on week-days between 9:30 A.M. and 1 P.M. (EST) to answer questions about legal rights. Pursues equality for women and girls through litigation, education, and public information programs.

On the Front Lines: Spiritual Healing

Inside the sprawling compound of the 10,000-member Faithful Central Bible Church in Inglewood, California, Mary Alice Haye, one of its several pastors, leads the counseling ministries as if they were a major business enterprise. But here, of course, all business is done in the name of God. Among the eighty to one hundred ministries is one especially for women, led by women. Healing for Damaged Emotions is twelve weeks of intensive group counseling, providing a powerful mix of mental, emotional, and spiritual well-being that is critical to so many of us. One subject that emerges regularly among the talk of relationship problems, work drama, and family issues is sexual abuse. Healing for Damaged Emotions is so popular that when Pastor Haye posted a bulletin six years ago to generate interest, 120 women showed up. Now Faithful Central offers eight to ten concurrent sessions, serving eight to ten women each. "We were overwhelmed with the number of believers who were struggling with things like anger and forgiveness," says Haye, who anchors the program with the spiritual self-help book *Healing for Damaged Emotions*, by David A. Seamands. "Here, women are challenged to work through their damage using Christ as a center. We organize the groups based on common themes, like age, or those with young children. Then we pray on it, and decide not only what group to put them in, but also which counselor to match them up with, based on the counselor's skills and spiritual maturity." The lay counselors, known as Encouragers, undergo seven months of training in spiritual counseling, followed by an apprenticeship, before they can lead their own group. In the sessions, faith, honesty, and confidentiality are musts. After three months of Christian fellowship and healing, many women emerge with lifelong connections, a deeper relationship with God, and a new sense of purpose. "It's just amazing to watch their victory," Haye says.

REFERRALS

Rape, Abuse & Incest National Network
635B Pennsylvania Avenue SE
Washington, DC 20003
(202) 544-1034, ext. 1
(800) 656-HOPE; (800) 656-4673
www.rainn.org

An organization that offers twenty-four-hour crisis intervention online and by phone. Can refer you to a nearby rape crisis center.

Association of Black Psychologists
P.O. Box 55999
Washington, DC 20040-5999
(202) 722-0808
www.abpsi.org
E-mail: admin@abpsi.org

An organization of professionals united to address the problems facing Black psychologists and the larger Black community. Web site provides a national listing of Black psychologists.

VOICES in Action, Inc. (Victims of Incest Can Emerge Survivors)
8041 Hosbrook, Suite 236
Cincinnati, OH 45236
(800) 7-VOICE-8; (800) 786-4238
www.voices-action.org
E-mail: voicesinaction@aol.com

Members can join their special interest groups, networks of survivors who have experienced similar types of abuse, backgrounds, or aftereffects.

National Organization for Victim Assistance
1730 Park Road NW
Washington, DC 20010
(202) 232-6682

(800) TRY NOVA; (800) 879-6682 for referrals to community-based victim assistance programs

www.trynova.org

The organization of victim and witness assistance programs and practitioners, criminal justice agencies and professionals, mental health professionals, researchers, former victims, and survivors that aims to promote rights and services for victims of crime and crisis.

National Mental Health Association

2001 N. Beauregard Street, 12th Floor

Alexandria, VA 22311

(800) 969-6642

www.nmha.org

The organization provides referrals to community mental health services.

American Art Therapy Association

1202 Allanson Road

Mundelein, IL 60060-3808

888-290-0878

www.arttherapy.org

Web site links to state chapters, which can provide information about local therapists.

American Dance Therapy Association

2000 Century Plaza, Suite 108

Columbia, MD 21044-3263

(410) 997-4040

www.adta.org

The membership organization for dance therapists nationwide provides links to local members.

American Society of Clinical Hypnosis

140 N. Bloomingdale Road

Bloomingdale, IL 60108-1017

(630) 980-4740
www.asch.net

The organization for health professionals who use hypnosis. Provides referrals through www.asch.net/referrals.asp.

American Music Therapy Association
8455 Colesville Road, Suite 1000
Silver Spring, MD 20910
(301) 589-3300
www.musictherapy.org

Advances the therapeutic use of music in rehabilitation. Provides referrals to music therapists via findMT@musictherapy.org.

EMDR (Eye Movement Desensitization and Reprocessing) Institute
EMDR Institute, Inc.
P.O. Box 750
Watsonville, CA 95077
(831) 372-3900
www.emdr.com

Web site provides listing of professionals trained to administer EMDR.

International Association of Reiki Professionals
P.O. Box 104
Harrisville, N.H. 03450
(603) 827-3290
www.iarp.org

Web site provides referrals at www.iarp.org/referral.html.

RESEARCH / PROFESSIONAL SUPPORT

National Sexual Violence Resource Center
123 N. Enola Drive
Enola, PA 17025
(717) 909-0710; (877) 739-3895

On the Front Lines: A Word Against Rape

First Aishah Shahidah Simmons got angry about the silence surrounding the rape of Black women and girls. Then she did something about it. That something is *NO!*, an acclaimed documentary that has been traveling the country for years now. "I started thinking about *NO!* in 1992," says Simmons, thirty-four, a Philadelphia writer, lecturer, and filmmaker, "when the Black clergy and prominent Black men were supporting Mike Tyson [in his trial for the rape of Desiree Washington], that was the beginning. I remembered many of those same men had supported Tawana Brawley [the upstate New York teenager who accused five White law enforcement officers of raping her]. So I started thinking, 'Oh, okay, so if White men rape us then we need to be outraged. But, if a prominent Black man is accused of or convicted of rape, then we're not supposed to talk about it.'" Once she began developing the film in 1994, Simmons envisioned a fifteen- or twenty-minute film, a statement of her outrage. It now tops eighty minutes, and she's still got more to say. Her decade-long odyssey in search of funding to complete the project shows that her message is not always well received. "Many Black people said this was like airing dirty laundry. In one grant rejection letter, they said, 'The fact can't be denied that a moral point of view in the Black community is that a woman shouldn't be in a man's room at 2 in the morning.' That was very painful." Simmons has pressed on, taking her rough cut from city to city, campus to campus, raising awareness and winning support from a broad cross section of Black activists, scholars, artists, and thinkers. The film, which is a mix of history (from a Black woman's perspective, of course), survivor testimonials, social criticism, music, dance, and spoken word, is destined for college campuses, community centers, and churches. It is a must-see for women and men of all socioeconomic backgrounds. "As African Americans, we are also affected by the stereotypes," Simmons says. "People think only people who really are dysfunctional perpetuate violence—not people who are 'successful.' I was raped in college. This is to say that this happens everywhere."

TTY: (717) 909-0715
www.nsvrc.org

The organization works with outside researchers to provide advocates with current information on various topics related to sexual violence.

American Professional Society on the Abuse of Children
APSAC National Office
P.O. Box 26901, CHO 3B-3406
Oklahoma City, OK 73190
(405) 271-8202
www.apsac.org

This national organization focuses on meeting the needs of professionals engaged in all aspects of services for maltreated children and their families.

Crimes Against Children Research Center
University of New Hampshire
20 College Road
#126 Horton Social Science Center
Durham, NH 03824
(603) 862-1888
www.unh.edu/ccrc

The center deals with the victimization of children and adolescents within and outside the family.

RELIGION-BASED SUPPORT

Center for the Prevention of Sexual and Domestic Violence
2400 N. 45th Street, #10
Seattle, WA 98103
(206) 634-1903
www.cpsdv.org

This interdenominational training and education center engages religious leaders to combat sexual and domestic abuse.

SASSY, Inc.
P.O. Box 727
Rice Lake, WI 54868
(715) 234-8445
www.sassyinc.org

This Christian/spiritual sexual and domestic violence support program promotes social changes needed to end sexual and domestic violence.

HELP FOR MEN

Male Survivor: The National Organization Against Male Sexual Victimization
PMB 103, 5505
Connecticut Avenue NW
Washington, DC 20015
(800) 738-4181
www.malesurvivor.org

National organization committed to preventing, healing, and eliminating sexual victimization of boys and men through treatment, research, education, advocacy, and activism. Includes a listing of mental health professionals offering their services to male survivors.

STATE COALITIONS

Their individual missions vary, but most state coalitions are networks of individuals and organizations working together to deliver education, support, and advocacy on sexual assault issues to survivors, service providers, and the public in general. Many coalitions provide referrals to community-based organizations for services like victim assistance and counseling and can refer you to local services geared to African Americans. Many lobby for changes in laws to improve the investigation and prosecution of sexual violence.

Alabama

Alabama Coalition Against Rape
207 Montgomery Street
P.O. Box 4091
Montgomery, AL 36104
(334) 264-0123
(888) 725-RAPE (7273)
www.acar.org

Alaska

Alaska Network on Domestic Violence and Sexual Assault
130 Seward Street, Room 209
Juneau, AK 99801
(907) 586-3650
(800) 520-2666
www.andvsa.org

Arizona

Arizona Sexual Assault Network
77 E. Thomas Road, Suite 110
Phoenix, AZ 85012
(602) 258-1195
www.azsan.org

Arkansas

Arkansas Coalition Against Sexual Assault
215 N. East Avenue
Fayetteville, AR 72701
(479) 527-0900
(866) 63-ACASA; (866) 632-2272
www.acasa.ws

California

California Coalition Against Sexual Assault
1215 K Street, Suite 1100
Sacramento, CA 95814
(916) 446-2520
www.calcasa.org

Colorado
Colorado Coalition Against Sexual Assault
1600 Downing Street, Suite 400
Denver, CO 80218
(303) 861-7033
(877) 37-CCASA; (877) 372-2272
www.ccasa.org

Connecticut
Connecticut Sexual Assault Crisis Services, Inc.
96 Pitkin Street
East Hartford, CT 06108
(860) 282-9881
(888) 999-5545
www.connsacs.org

Delaware
CONTACT Delaware
P.O. Box 9525
Wilmington, DE 19809
(302) 761-9800
www.contactdelaware.org

DC
D.C. Rape Crisis Center
P.O. Box 34125
Washington, DC 20043
(202) 232-0789
www.dcrcc.org

Florida
Florida Council Against Sexual Violence
1311A Paul Russell Road, Suite 204
Tallahassee, FL 32301
(850) 297-2000
(888) 956-7273
www.fcasv.org

Georgia
Georgia Network to End Sexual Assault
619 Edgewood Avenue SE, Suite 104
Atlanta, GA 30312
(678) 701-2700
(800) 656-4673
www.gnesa.org

Hawaii
Hawaii Coalition Against Sexual Assault
741A Sunset Avenue, Room 105
Honolulu, HI 96816
(808) 733-9038
E-mail: msshari@aloha.net

Idaho
Idaho Coalition Against Sexual and Domestic Violence
815 Park Boulevard, Suite 140
Boise, ID 83712
(208) 384-0419
(888) 293-6118
www.idvsa.org

Illinois
Illinois Coalition Against Sexual Assault
100 N. 16th Street
Springfield, IL 62703
(217) 753-4117
www.icasa.org

Indiana
Indiana Coalition Against Sexual Assault
55 Monument Circle, Suite 1224
Indianapolis, IN 46204
(317) 423-0233
(800) 691-2272
www.incasa.org

Iowa

Iowa Coalition Against Sexual Assault
2603 Bell Avenue, Suite 102
Des Moines, IA 50321
(515) 244-7424
www.iowacasa.org

Kansas

Kansas Coalition Against Sexual and Domestic Violence
220 SW 33rd Street, Suite 100
Topeka, KS 66611
(785) 232-9784
www.kcsdv.org

Kentucky

Kentucky Association of Sexual Assault Programs, Inc.
106A St. James Court
Frankfort, KY 40601
(502) 226-2704
(800) 656-4673
www.kasap.org

Louisiana

Louisiana Foundation Against Sexual Assault
P.O. Box 40
Independence, LA 70443
(985) 345-5995
(888) 995-7273
http://lafasa.org

Maine

Maine Coalition Against Sexual Assault
83 Western Avenue, Suite 2
Augusta, ME 04330
(207) 626-0034
www.mecasa.org

Maryland
Maryland Coalition Against Sexual Assault, Inc.
1517 Gov. Ritchie Highway, Suite 207
Arnold, MD 21012
(410) 974-4507
(800) 983-7273
www.mcasa.org

Massachusetts
Jane Doe, Inc.: Massachusetts Coalition Against Sexual Assault and Domestic Violence
14 Beacon Street, Suite 507
Boston, MA 02108
(617) 248-0922
(877) 785-2020
www.janedoe.org

Michigan
Michigan Coalition Against Domestic and Sexual Violence
3893 Okemos Road, Suite B2
Okemos, MI 48864
(517) 347-7000
www.mcadsv.org

Minnesota
Minnesota Coalition Against Sexual Assault
420 N. Fifth Street, Suite 690
Minneapolis, MN 55401
(612) 313-2797
(800) 964-8847
www.mncasa.org

Mississippi
Mississippi Coalition Against Sexual Assault
510 George Street
Jackson, MS 39201
(601) 948-0555
(888) 987-9011
www.mscasa.org

Missouri
Missouri Coalition Against Sexual Assault
1000-D Northeast Drive
Jefferson City, MO 65109
(573) 636-8776
www.mocasa.missouri.org

Montana
Montana Coalition Against Domestic and Sexual Violence
32 South Ewing
Helena, MT 59601
(406) 443-7794
www.mcadsv.com

Nebraska
Nebraska Domestic Violence Sexual Assault Coalition
825 M Street, Suite 404
Lincoln, NE 68508
(402) 476-6256
www.ndvsac.org

Nevada
Nevada Coalition Against Sexual Violence
3027 E. Sunset Road, Suite 101
Las Vegas, NV 89120
(702) 940-2033
Fax (702) 940-2032
www.ncasv.org

New Hampshire
New Hampshire Coalition Against Domestic and Sexual Violence
4 S. State Street
Concord, NH 03301
(603) 224-8893
(800) 277-5570
(800) 735-2964
www.nhcadsv.org

New Jersey
New Jersey Coalition Against Sexual Assault
2333 Whitehorse Mercerville Road, Suite B
Trenton, NJ 08619
(609) 631-4450
(800) 601-7200 (24-hour hotline)
www.njcasa.org

New Mexico
New Mexico Coalition of Sexual Abuse Programs
3909 Juan Tabo Boulevard, Suite 6
Albuquerque, NM 87111
(505) 883-8020
www.swcp.com/nmcsaas

New York
New York State Coalition Against Sexual Assault
63 Colvin Avenue
Albany, NY 12206
(518) 482-4222
www.nyscasa.org

North Carolina
North Carolina Coalition Against Sexual Assault
4426 Louisburg Road, Suite 100
Raleigh, NC 27616
(919) 431-0995
(888) 737-2272
www.nccasa.org

North Dakota
North Dakota Council on Abused Women's Services / Coalition Against Sexual
    Assault in North Dakota
418 E. Rosser Avenue, #320
Bismarck, ND 58501
(701) 255-6240
(888) 255-6240
www.ndcaws.org

Ohio
Ohio Coalition on Sexual Assault
933 N. High Street, Suite 120B
Worthington, OH 43085
(614) 268-3322
www.ocosa.org

Oklahoma
Oklahoma Coalition Against Domestic Violence and Sexual Assault
2525 NW Express Way, Suite 101
Oklahoma City, OK 73112
(405) 848-1815
www.ocadvsa.org

Oregon
Oregon Coalition Against Domestic and Sexual Violence
115 Mission Street SE, Suite 100
Salem, OR 97302
(503) 365-9644
www.ocadsv.com

Pennsylvania
Pennsylvania Coalition Against Rape
125 N. Enola Drive
Enola, PA 17025
(717) 728-9740
(888) 772-PCAR; (888- 772-7227)
www.pcar.org

Rhode Island
Sexual Assault and Trauma Resource Center of Rhode Island
300 Richmond Street, Suite 205
Providence, RI 02903
(401) 421-4100
www.satrc.org

South Carolina
South Carolina Coalition Against Domestic Violence and Sexual Assault
1320 Richland Street
Columbia, SC 29202
(803) 256-2900
(800) 260-9293
www.sccadvasa.org

South Dakota
South Dakota Coalition Against Domestic Violence and Sexual Assault
106 Capital Avenue
Pierre, SD 57501
(605) 945-0869
(800) 572-9196
www.southdakotacoalition.org

Tennessee
Tennessee Coalition Against Domestic and Sexual Violence
P.O. Box 120972
Nashville, TN 37212
(615) 386-9406
(800) 289-9018
www.tcadsv.org

Texas
Texas Association Against Sexual Assault
7701 N. Lamar Boulevard, Suite 200
Austin, TX 78752
(512) 474-7190
www.taasa.org

Utah
Utah Coalition Against Sexual Assault
4 W. 400 North
Salt Lake City, UT 84111
(801) 746-0404
www.ucasa.org

Vermont
Vermont Network Against Domestic Violence and Sexual Assault
P.O. Box 405
Montpelier, VT 05601
(802) 223-1302
(800) 489-7273 (24-hour hotline)
www.vtnetwork.org

Virginia
Virginians Aligned Against Sexual Assault
508 Dale Avenue
Charlottesville, VA 22903
(434) 979-9002
(800) 838-8238
www.vaasa.org

Washington
Washington Coalition of Sexual Assault Programs
2415 Pacific Avenue, SE
Olympia, WA 98501
(360) 754-7583
www.wcsap.org

West Virginia
West Virginia Foundation for Rape Information and Services, Inc.
112 Braddock Street
Fairmont, WV 26554
(304) 366-9500
www.fris.org

Wisconsin
Wisconsin Coalition Against Sexual Assault
600 Williamson Street, Suite N-2
Madison, WI 53703
(608) 257-1516
www.wcasa.org

Wyoming
Wyoming Coalition Against Domestic Violence and Sexual Assault
409 S. 4th Street
P.O. Box 236
Laramie, WY 82073
(307) 755-5481
(800) 990-3877
www.users.qwest.net/~wyomingcoalition/index.htm

HELP FOR OFFENDERS

STOP IT NOW!
P.O. Box 495
Haydenville, MA 01039
(413) 268-3096
(888) PREVENT; (888-773-8368)
www.stopitnow.org

This nonprofit organization encourages abusers and potential abusers to stop and seek help and increases public awareness of the trauma of child sexual abuse. Offers treatment referrals for offenders and potential offenders.

The Safer Society Foundation, Inc., Sexual Abuser Treatment Referral Line
PO Box 340
Brandon, VT 05733-0340
(802) 247-3132 (Monday through Friday, 9 A.M.–4:30 P.M., Eastern time)
Requests for referrals may be faxed: (802) 247-4233
To e-mail request: tammyk@sover.net.
www.safersociety.org

National Adolescent Perpetration Network
Kempe Children's Center
1825 Marion Street
Denver, CO 80218
(303) 864-5192
To e-mail request for referral: Ryan.Gail@tchden.org
www.kempecenter.org

On the Front Lines: From One to Many

Charlene Walker just knew that she wasn't the only sister in the St. Louis area struggling with issues related to having been sexually abused by a relative when she was a little girl. So in October 2000, Walker, who works as executive assistant to Donald Suggs, publisher of the *St. Louis American,* a Black weekly, started a nonprofit organization to help Black women survivors come together. She began by explaining her mission to friends and coworkers. Her group, Victims to Victors, has slowly grown by word of mouth, inspired by a regular newsletter, *The Triumphant,* which she mails to about sixty people. Walker infuses her newsletters with health information, support group activities, recommended books, Web sites and conferences, and spiritual encouragement. Walker, who sees herself as "a beacon of light for survivors," says she established Victims to Victors particularly for women who may not find their churches responsive to their needs. "Our purpose is to bless and thus be blessed by empowering survivors to reach their 'divine destiny,'" her mission statement reads. Members stay in touch by phone or e-mail, responding to newsletter topics and passing on information of their own. Walker's vision includes monthly meetings and an annual conference where Black women come from across the country to connect, exchange information, and heal. She has become recognized as a local authority on child sexual abuse, conducting domestic violence workshops for church and community groups, and providing her expertise to local media. She exemplifies the power of just one person to change people's lives. "I do a little bit every day," she says, "but I see so much in the future, here in St. Louis, throughout the state, and the country. The possibilities are endless."

The network of professionals works with sexually abusive youth. Provides information and referrals.

Child Molestation Research & Prevention Institute
1100 Piedmont Avenue, Suite 2
Atlanta, GA 30309
(404) 872-5152

or

P.O. Box 27160

Oakland, CA 94602

(510) 530-7980

www.childmolestationprevention.org

This national organization is dedicated to preventing child sexual abuse through research, education, and family support. Includes a national list of therapists who evaluate and treat children, teenagers, and adults who are at risk for developing or who have a sexual interest in children.

Mustard Seed Counseling Services

111 Court Street, Suite 2L

Brooklyn, NY 11201

(718) 875-7411

mustardseed1420@aol.com

An agency that provides counseling services for adult and adolescent sexual abusers and non-offending parents in the New York City area.

The Association for the Treatment of Sexual Abusers

4900 S.W. Griffith Drive, Suite 274

Beaverton, OR 97005

(503) 643-1023

www.atsa.com

The nonprofit international organization focuses on the prevention of sexual abuse through effective management of sex offenders. Provides referrals to affiliated treatment centers.

Sex Abuse Treatment Alliance

P.O. Box 1191

Okemos, MI 48805

(517) 482-2085

The nonprofit organization works to prevent sexual abuse by educating the public and supporting and working with those who have abused and who have been abused. Provides a network of support for abusers who are currently in treatment and for those in prison.

Center for Sex Offender Management
8403 Colesville Road, Suite 720
Silver Spring, MD 20910
(301) 589-9383
www.csom.org

This program of the Office of Justice Programs, U.S. Department of Justice, aims to improve the management of adult and juvenile sex offenders. Provides technical assistance and training to those who treat and supervise offenders.

BOOKS

These works of nonfiction and fiction are recommended reading for survivors of child sexual abuse:

Ainscough, Carolyn, and Kay Toon. *Breaking Free: A Self-Help Guide for Adults Who Were Sexually Abused as Children*. Fisher Books, Tucson, 1993.

Allison, Dorothy. *Bastard Out of Carolina*. Dutton Book/Penguin Group, New York, 1992.

Angelou, Maya. *I Know Why the Caged Bird Sings*. Bantam, New York, 1983 (reissue).

Avery, Byllye. *An Altar of Words*. Broadway Books, New York, 1998.

Bass, Ellen, and Laura Davis. *The Courage to Heal: A Guide for Women Survivors of Child Sexual Abuse*. Third edition. Harper Perennial, New York, 1994.

Blume, E. Sue. *Secret Survivors: Uncovering Incest and Its Aftereffects in Women*. Ballantine Books, New York, 1990.

Bynum, Juanita. *No More Sheets: The Truth About Sex*. Pneuma Life Publishing, Lanham, Maryland, 2000.

Cole, Johnnetta Betsch, and Beverly Guy-Sheftall. *Gender Talk: The Struggle for Women's Equality in African American Communities*. Ballantine Books, New York, 2003.

Coleman, Monica A. *The Dinah Project: A Handbook for Congregational Response to Sexual Violence*. Pilgrim Press, Berea, Ohio, 2004.

Conroy, Pat. *The Prince of Tides*. Houghton Mifflin, New York, 1986.

Crinch, Joseph E., and Kimberly A. Crinch. *Shifting the Burden of Truth: Suing Child Sexual Abusers—A Legal Guide for Survivors and Their Supporters*. Recollex Publishing, Lake Oswego, Oregon, 1992.

Davis, Laura. *I Thought We'd Never Speak Again: The Road from Estrangement to Reconciliation*. HarperCollins, New York, 2002.

Dugan, Meg Kennedy, and Roger Hock. *It's My Life Now: Starting Over After an Abusive Relationship or Domestic Violence*. Routledge, New York, 2000.

Fisher, Antwone Q. *Finding Fish*. HarperTorch, New York, 2002.

Guy-Sheftall, Beverly. *Words of Fire: An Anthology of African-American Feminist Thought*. New Press, New York, 1995.

Hollies, Linda H., *Taking Back My Yesterdays: Lessons in Forgiving and Moving Forward with Your Life*. The Pilgrim Press, Cleveland, 1977.

hooks, bell. *Ain't I a Woman: Black Women and Feminism*. South End Press, Boston, 1992 (reissue).

Kashef, Ziba. *Like a Natural Woman: The Black Woman's Guide to Alternative Healing*. Kensington Publishing Corp., New York, 2001.

Lew, Mike. *Victims No Longer: Men Recovering from Incest and Other Sexual Child Abuse*. HarperCollins, New York, 1986.

Lockhart, Zelda. *Fifth Born*. Atria Books, New York, 2002.

McClurkin, Donnie. *Eternal Victim, Eternal Victor*. Pneuma Life Publishing, Lanham, Maryland, 2001.

Morrison, Toni. *The Bluest Eye*. Plume, New York, 1994 (reissue).

Pierce-Baker, Charlotte. *Surviving the Silence: Black Women's Stories of Rape*. W. W. Norton and Co., New York, 1998.

Richardson, Brenda, and Brenda Wade. *What Mama Couldn't Tell Us About Love: Healing the Emotional Legacy of Racism by Celebrating Our Light*. Perennial, New York, 2000.

Robinson, Lori S. *I Will Survive: The African-American Guide to Healing from Sexual Assault and Abuse*. Seal Press, New York, 2002.

Rose, Tricia. *Longing to Tell: Black Women Talk About Sexuality and Intimacy.* Farrar, Straus and Giroux, New York, 2003.

Sapphire. *Push.* Vintage Books, New York, 1997.

Seamands, David A. *Healing for Damaged Emotions.* Chariot Victor Books, Colorado Springs, 1991.

Shange, Ntozake. *For Colored Girls Who Have Considered Suicide, When the Rainbow Is Enuf.* Scribner, New York, 1997 (reissue).

Singleton, D. Kim. *Broken Silence: Opening Your Heart and Mind to Therapy: A Black Woman's Recovery Guide.* One World/Strivers Row, New York, 2003.

Vanzant, Iyanla. *Yesterday, I Cried.* Fireside, New York, 2000.

Walker, Alice. *The Color Purple.* Harcourt Brace Jovanovich, New York, 1982.

Wallace, Michele. *Black Macho and the Myth of the Superwoman.* Warner Books, New York, 1983 (reissue).

West, Carolyn M. *Violence in the Lives of Black Women: Battered, Black, and Blue.* The Haworth Press, Binghamton, New York, 2003.

West, Traci C. *Wounds of the Spirit.* New York University Press, New York, 1999.

White, Evelyn C. *The Black Women's Health Book: Speaking for Ourselves.* Seal Press, Seattle, 1990.

Wyatt, Gail E. *Stolen Women.* John Wiley & Sons, Inc., New York, 1997.

Chapter One: Was It Sexual Abuse?

1 The compulsion to engage children in a sexual manner has been identified as a mental impairment, pedophilia, according to the American Psychiatric Association's *Diagnostic and Statistical Manual of Mental Disorders,
Fourth Edition*. The DSM-IV says a person meets the criteria for pedophilia
if they have "over a period of at least six months, recurrent, intense sexually arousing fantasies, sexual urges, or behaviors involving sexual activity with a prepubescent child or children (generally age thirteen or
younger)." Under the DSM-IV criteria, a pedophile is at least sixteen
years old with a sexual interest in someone at least five years younger. Sex
play between children of the same age, such as "playing doctor," is considered normal. But some sexual behavior is considered problematic when
it occurs frequently or in secrecy, between children of significantly different ages or developmental abilities, when it is associated with emotional distress or occurs under coercion or force, according to the
National Center on Sexual Behavior of Youth. A person can be a
pedophile but not a sexual abuser. They cross the line once they act on
their impulses. While some pedophiles are attracted only to children,
others are also attracted to and have sexual relationships with adults.

2. Howard N. Snyder, "Sexual Assault of Young Children as Reported to
Law Enforcement," National Center for Juvenile Justice (2000). Sixty-
seven percent of all victims of sexual assault reported to law enforcement agencies were juvenile (under age eighteen), and one in seven
victims were under age six; 34.2 percent of juvenile victims were abused
by a family member and 58.7 percent were abused by an acquaintance.

3. Snyder, "Sexual Assault of Young Children as Reported to Law Enforcement." Females make up 86 percent of all sexual assault victims under age
eighteen; 95 percent of sexual abuse of girls and 80 percent of sexual abuse
of boys is committed by men.

4. Traci C. West, *Wounds of the Spirit: Black Women, Violence and Resistance Ethics* (New York: New York University Press, 1999), p. 5.

5. L. Miriam Dickinson, Frank Verloin deGruy III, W. Perry Dickinson, and Lucy M. Candib, "Health-Related Quality of Life and Symptom Profiles of Female Survivors of Sexual Abuse," *Journal of the American Medical Association* 8 (1999): pp. 35–43.

6. Timothy C. Hart and Callie Rennison, "Reporting Crime to the Police, 1992–2000," Bureau of Justice Statistics. According to an analysis of the National Crime Victimization Survey, rape/sexual assault was reported only about 31 percent of the time, compared with aggravated assault (55 percent) and simple assault (38 percent). Rennison, "Rape and Sexual Assault: Reporting to Police and Medical Attention, 1992–2000." This analysis showed that 26 percent of sexual assaults of females were not reported. Sexual assault was most often *not* reported because it was deemed a "personal" matter, the studies showed.

7. Various studies of adults looking back on their childhoods have found numbers ranging from 15 to 33 percent of females and 13 to 16 percent of males who report being sexually abused in childhood, according to M. A. Polusny and V. M. Follette, "Long Term Correlates of Child Sexual Abuse: Theory and Review of Empirical Literature," *Applied and Preventive Psychology* 4 (1995): pp. 143–66, and Jim Hopper, "Sexual Abuse of Males: Prevalence and Lasting Effects and Resources," 1997. Hopper, a research associate at the Boston University School of Medicine, maintains an extensive Web site on sexual abuse, including a thoughtful section on statistics and research: www.jimhopper.com.

8. Based on U.S. Census 2000 figures: African Americans eighteen and older; www.census.gov/population/cen2000/phc-t108/tab03.xls.

9. Victimization rates are based on the number of cases of reported abuse: National Child Abuse and Neglect Data System, 2000, Administration on Children, Youth and Families, U.S. Department of Health and Human Services. Severity of abuse: Diana Russell et al., "The Long-Term Effects of Incestuous Abuse: A Comparison of African American and White American Victims," in Gail E. Wyatt and Gloria Johnson Powell, eds., *Lasting Effects of Child Sexual Abuse* (Newbury Park, CA: Sage Publications, 1988), p. 129.

10. Bureau of Justice Statistics: Sexual Assault of Young Children as Reported to Law Enforcement, 2000.

11. Third National Incidence Study of Child Sexual Abuse and Neglect, National Center on Child Abuse and Neglect, U.S. Department of Health and Human Services, September 1996.

12. Gail E. Wyatt et al., UCLA/Drew Women & Family Project study, reported in the *American Journal of Public Health,* April 2002.

13. E. Sue Blume, *Secret Survivors: Uncovering Incest and Its AftereVects in Women* (NewYork: Ballantine Books, 1991), p. 12.

14. Stephanie Doyle Peters, "Child Sexual Abuse and Later Psychological Problems," in Gail E. Wyatt and Gloria Johnson Powell, eds., *Lasting Effects of Child Sexual Abuse* (Newbury Park, California: Sage Publications, 1988), p. 112.

15. Debra Boyer and David Fine, "Sexual Abuse as a Factor in Adolescent Pregnancy and Child Maltreatment," *Family Planning Perspectives,* 24 (1992): pp. 4–11, 19.

16. Mimi Silbert, "Treatment of Prostitution Victims of Sexual Abuse," in Irving Stuart and Joanne Greer, eds., *Victims of Sexual Aggression* (NewYork: Van Nostrand Reinhold, 1984).

17. Wyatt et al., UCLA/Drew University Women and Family Project study.

18. Third National Incidence Study of Child Sexual Abuse and Neglect.

19. Russell, et. al., "The Long-Term Effects of Incestuous Abuse," p. 131.

20. Gail E. Wyatt, "Sociocultural Context of African American and White American Women's Rape," *Journal of Social Issues* 48 (1992): pp. 77–91.

21. Russell, et. al., "The Long-Term Effects of Incestuous Abuse," p. 131.

22. Ibid., p. 114.

23. In *Penny Penguin's Secret,* Willie Mae Anthony's excellent children's book on childhood sexual abuse, Penny's parents tell Uncle Peter Penguin how much he had hurt Penny and "that he had broken the family trust." "When Penny found out that Uncle Peter Penguin was no longer welcomed in their home she was very happy to know that her family still loved her." The book is published by Million Words Publishing, P.O. Box 286281, St. Louis, MO 63136.

24. Denise Cara Dabney, "Resilient Women: Childhood Sexual Abuse of African American Women and Their Coping and Healing," Ph.D. dissertation, Brandeis University [2000], p. 39.

25. Meg Kennedy Dugan and Roger R. Hock, *It's My Life Now: Starting Over After an Abusive Relationship or Domestic Violence* (NewYork: Routledge, 2000), pp. 35–38.

26. Ibid., p. 36.

27. West, *Wounds of the Spirit,* pp. 73–74.

28. Ibid., p. 109.

29. Kennedy Dugan and Hock, *It's My Life Now: Starting Over After an Abusive Relationship or Domestic Violence,* p. 39.

30. Brenda Richardson and Brenda Wade, *What Mama Couldn't Tell Us About Love: Healing the Emotional Legacy of Racism by Celebrating Our Light* (New York: Perennial, 2000), pp. xix–xx.

31. Gail E. Wyatt, *Stolen Women: Reclaiming Our Sexuality, Taking Back Our Lives* (New York: John Wiley & Sons, 1997), pp. 22–23.

32. Ibid.

33. Deborah Gray White, *Ar'n't I a Woman: Female Slaves in the Plantation South* (New York: W. W. Norton, 1999), p. 68.

34. Ibid., pp. 32–33.

35. Audrey Edwards, "Black and White Women: What Still Divides Us?" *Essence,* March 1993, p. 77.

36. Nancy Boyd-Franklin, *Black Families in Therapy: A Multisystems Approach* (New York: The Guilford Press, 1989), p. 16.

37. Ibid., p 8.

38. Ibid., pp. 160–61.

Chapter Two: Overcoming Fear and Shame

1. David Finkelhor et al., *A Sourcebook on Child Sexual Abuse* (Beverly Hills: Sage Publications, 1986), pp. 181–85.

2. Gail E. Wyatt, Michael D. Newcomb, and Monika H. Riederle, *Sexual Abuse and Consensual Sex: Women's Developmental Patterns and Outcomes* (Newbury Park, CA: Sage Publications, 1993), p. 43.

3. Traci C. West, *Wounds of the Spirit: Black Women, Violence and Resistance Ethics* (New York: New York University Press, 1999), p. 67.

4. Carolyn Ainscough and Kay Toon, *Breaking Free: A Self-Help Guide for Adults Who Were Sexually Abused as Children* (Tucson: Fisher Books, 1993), p. 33.

5. Many of the effects listed are outlined in *Sexual Abuse and Consensual Sex: Women's Developmental Patterns and Outcomes* and *Breaking Free: A Self-Help Guide for Adults Who Were Sexually Abused as Children*; others come from the National Center for Victims of Crime, www.ncvc.org.

6. West, *Wounds of the Spirit,* p. 17.

7. Ainscough and Toon, *Breaking Free,* p. 45.

Chapter Three: Family Matters

1. Aphrodite Matsakis, *I Can't Get Over It: A Handbook for Trauma Survivors,* 2nd ed. (Oakland: New Harbinger Publications, 1996), p. 292. Matsakis writes, "The horror of being a victim of family violence is that you are being hurt by someone who claims to love you or who has promised or is obligated to take care of you."

2. Diana Russell, et al., "The Long-Term Effects of Incestuous Abuse: A Comparison of Afro-American and White-American Victims," in Gail E. Wyatt and Gloria Johnson Powell, eds., *Lasting Effects of Child Sexual Abuse* (Newbury Park, CA: Sage Publications, 1988), p. 128.

3. Ibid., p. 127.

4. Ibid., pp. 127, 129.

5. Nancy Boyd-Franklin, *Black Families in Therapy: A Multisystems Approach* (New York: The Guilford Press, 1989), p. 14.

6. Ibid., p. 15.

7. Ellen Bass and Laura Davis, *The Courage to Heal,* 3rd ed. (New York: Harper Perennial, 1994), p. 105.

8. Boyd-Franklin, *Black Families in Therapy,* p. 21.

Chapter Four: "Getting It Out" and Healing

1. Karen Scott Collins, Cathy Schoen, Susan Joseph, Lisa Duchon, Elisabeth Simantov, and Michele Yellowitz, "The Commonwealth Fund 1998 Survey of Women's Health," Commonwealth Foundation.

2. Ibid.

3. Ibid.

4. Ibid.

5. Ibid.

6. National Institute of Mental Health, www.nimh.gov/publicat/depemployee.cfm#link1.

7. Cecilia Capuzzi Simon, "A Change of Mind," *The Washington Post,* Sept. 3, 2002.

8. Jill M. Scrafin, "Treating Disrupted Relationships: Couples Therapy for Female Child Sexual Abuse Survivors and Their Partners," *National Center for Post Traumatic Stress Disorder Clinical Quarterly,* 6 (1996): pp. 42–45.

9. Compiled from social worker Maelinda Turner, the organization Victims of Incest Can Emerge Survivors (VOICES), and Ellen Bass and Laura

Davis, *The Courage to Heal: A Guide for Women Survivors of Child Sexual Abuse* (New York: Harper Perennial, 1994).

10. American Dance Therapy Association, www.adta.org; cited May 18, 2003.

11. American Art Therapy Association, www.arttherapy.org; cited May 18, 2003.

12. American Music Therapy Association, www.musictherapy.org; cited May 18, 2003.

13. Francine Shapiro and Margot Silk Forrest, *EMDR: The Breakthrough "Eye Movement" Therapy for Overcoming Anxiety, Stress and Trauma* (New York: Basic Books, 1997), p. 6.

14. American Society of Clinical Hypnosis, www.asch.net; cited May 24, 2003. For referrals: www.asch.net/referrals.asp.

15. International Association of Reiki Professionals, www.iarp.org; cited May 18, 2003. To find practitioners: http://www.iarp.org/referral.html.

16. Educational Resources Information Center (ERIC), no. ED357333; sponsored by the U.S. Department of Education; http://www.ericfacility. net/ericdigests/ed357333.html.

17. Adapted from Thomas A. Parham, Joseph L. White, and Adisa Ajumu, *The Psychology of Blacks: An African-Centered Perspective,* 3rd ed. (Upper Saddle River, NJ: Prentice Hall, 2000). The authors write that Ma'at also defines "the five dimensions of the African character": divinity, teachability, perfectability, free will, and moral and social responsibility.

18. Malidoma Patrice Somé, *The Healing Wisdom of Africa: Finding Life Purpose Through Nature, Ritual and Community* (New York: J. P. Tarcher/Putnam), p. 191.

19. Ibid., p. 38.

Chapter Five: Protecting and Saving Our Children

1. Howard N. Snyder, "Sexual Assault of Young Children as Reported to Law Enforcement: Victim, Incident and Offender Characteristics," National Center for Juvenile Justice, 2000.

2. Ibid.

3. David Finkelhor et al., *Child Sexual Abuse: New Theory and Research* (New York: The Free Press, 1984), p. 138.

4. David Finkelhor and Larry Baron, "High-Risk Children," in David Finkelhor et al., *A Sourcebook on Child Sexual Abuse* (Beverly Hills: Sage Publications, 1986), p. 64.

5. Snyder, "Sexual Assault of Young Children as Reported to Law Enforcement."

6. M. Joycelyn Elders and Alexa E. Albert, "Adolescent Pregnancy and Sexual Abuse," JAMA Women's Health Information Center, *Journal of the American Medical Association* 280 (1998): pp. 648–49.

7. David Finkelhor, *A Sourcebook on Child Sexual Abuse* (Beverly Hills, California: Sage Publications, 1986), p. 74.

8. Carole Jenny, Thomas A. Roesler, and Kimberly L. Poyer, "Are Children at Risk for Sexual Abuse by Homosexuals?" *Pediatrics* 94 (1994): 41–44. This study found that in 82 percent of cases of suspected child sexual abuse, the alleged offender was a heterosexual partner of a close relative of the child.

9. U.S. Department of Health and Human Services, Administration for Children and Families, http://nccanch.acf.hhs.gov/pubs/factsheets/about.cfm. The act has been amended several times, most recently in 2003.

10. Teena Sorenson and Barbara Snow, "How Children Tell: The Process of Disclosure in Sexual Abuse," *Child Welfare* 70 (1991): pp. 3–15. An analysis of substantiated cases of sexual abuse showed that 11 percent of children disclosed sexual abuse without denial in an initial investigative interview.

11. Finkelhor et al., *Child Sexual Abuse*, p. 54. Table 5-1 outlines preconditions and explores individual as well as social/cultural factors.

12. Douglas W. Pryor, *Unspeakable Acts: Why Men Sexually Abuse Children* (New York: New York University Press, 1996) p. 123.

13. Ibid., p. 145.

14. E. Sue Blume, *Secret Survivors: Uncovering Incest and Its Aftereffects in Women* (New York: Ballantine Books, 1991), p. 5. The author notes that this is sometimes called "covert" or "emotional" incest or seduction.

15. Pryor, *Unspeakable Acts*, p. 124.

16. Finkelhor et al., *Child Sexual Abuse*, p. 17. Finkelhor addresses the issue of whether children can consent to a sexual relationship: "Children may know that they like the adult, that the physical sensations feel good, and on this basis may make a choice. But they lack the knowledge the adult has about sex and what they are undertaking."

17. Gail E. Wyatt and Gloria Johnson Powell, *Lasting Effects of Child Sexual Abuse* (Newbury Park, CA: Sage Publications, 1988), p. 113. The authors note

that a lack of maternal warmth has been linked with mental health problems, including depression.

18. Finkelhor and Baron, "High-Risk Children," pp. 61–80, for first five factors, others cited by the experts I interviewed.

19. Finkelhor et al., *Child Sexual Abuse,* p. 28.

20. Snyder, "Sexual Assault of Young Children as Reported to Law Enforcement."

21. Adapted from "7 Steps to Protecting Children from Sexual Abuse: A Guide for Responsible Adults," with permission from Darkness to Light.

22. Adapted with permission from Good Touch/Bad Touch®.

Chapter Six: Helping Boys and Men

1. "Psychiatric Effects of Media Violence," American Psychiatric Association, www.psych.org/public_info/media_violence.cfm. Cited April 22, 2003.

2. Michael Eric Dyson, "Behind the Mask," *Essence,* November 1999, p. 108.

3. Stephen Donaldson, "Rape of Males," in Wayne R. Dynes, ed., *Encyclopedia of Homosexuality* (New York: Garland Publications, 1990), p. 1094.

4. Howard N. Snyder, "Sexual Assault of Young Children as Reported to Law Enforcement: Victim, Incident and Offender Characteristics," National Center for Juvenile Justice (2000).

5. Cathy Schoen, Karen Davis, Catherine DesRoches, and Alexander Shekhdar, "The Health of Adolescent Boys: Commonwealth Fund Survey Findings," 1997. Based on a survey of 3,586 girls and 3,162 boys. http://www.cmwf.org/programs/women/boysv271.asp.

6. Ibid.

7. Ibid.

8. Ibid.

9. Howard N. Snyder, "Sexual Assault of Young Children as Reported to Law Enforcement," National Center for Juvenile Justice (2000). Jim Hopper, "Sexual Abuse of Males: Prevalence and Lasting Effects and Resources," 1997.

10. Lawrence A. Greenfield, "Child Victimizers: Violent Offenders and Their Victims," Bureau of Justice Statistics, 1996.

11. William C. Holmes and Gail B. Slap, "Sexual Abuse of Boys," *Journal of the American Medical Association,* Dec. 2, 1998, pp. 1855–62.

12. Tamala Edwards, "Men Who Sleep with Men: Brothers on the Down Low Pose a Serious AIDS Risk to Black Women," *Essence,* October 2001.

13. Holmes and Slap, "Sexual Abuse of Boys."

14. Mike Lew, *Victims No Longer* (New York: HarperCollins, 1988), p. 55.

15. Holmes and Slap, "Sexual Abuse of Boys."

16. *Los Angeles Times* poll, July 1985.

17. Associated Press, Sept. 8, 2002.

18. Eli Newberger, *The Men They Will Become: The Nature and Nurture of Male Character* (New York: Perseus Publishing, 1999), p. 66.

19. Ellis Cose, *The Envy of the World: On Being a Black Man in America* (New York: Washington Square Press, 2002), p. 139.

20. Cathy S. Widom and Michael G. Maxfield, "An Update on the 'Cycle of Violence,'" National Institute of Justice, February 2001.

21. Snyder, "Sexual Assault of Young Children as Reported to Law Enforcement."

22. This information was compiled with the help of the Rosa Parks Sexual Assault Crisis Center in Los Angeles, and the National Organization Against Male Sexual Victimization (www.malesurvivor.org).

Chapter Seven: Challenging Abusers

1. David Finkelhor and Richard Omrod, "Child Abuse Reported to the Police," Office of Juvenile Justice and Delinquency Prevention, 2001. Kathleen Coulborn Miller and James Henry, "Child Sexual Abuse: A Case Study in Community Management," *Child Abuse and Neglect* 24 (2000): pp. 1215–1225.

2. David Finkelhor, *Child Sexual Abuse: New Theory and Research* (New York: The Free Press, 1984), p. 54. Table 5-1 outlines preconditions and explores individual as well as social/cultural factors.

3. American Psychiatric Association Fact Sheet on pedophilia, October 1997.

4. Howard N. Snyder, "Sexual Assault of Young Children as Reported to Law Enforcement: Victim, Incident and Offender Characteristics," National Center for Juvenile Justice (2000).

5. American Psychiatric Association Fact Sheet on pedophilia, October 1997.

6. Peter Finn, "Sex Offender Community Notification," National Institute of Justice, 1997. The number of sex offenders quadrupled from 1980 to 1994, increasing from 20,500 to 88,000.

7. Ibid.

8. Linda Villarosa, "To Prevent Sexual Abuse, Abusers Step Forward," *The New York Times*, December 3, 2002.

9. Lawrence A. Greenfeld, "Child Victimizers: Violent Offenders and Their Victims," Bureau of Justice Statistics, 1996.

10. Gene Abel et al., "Self-Reported Sex Crimes of Non-Incarcerated Paraphiliacs," *Journal of Interpersonal Violence,* 2 (1987): pp. 3–25.

11. National Center on the Sexual Behavior of Youth Fact Sheet: "What Research Shows about Adolescent Sex Offenders," Snyder, "Sexual Assault of Young Children as Reported to Law Enforcement."

12. Lawrence A. Greenfeld, "Sex Offenses and Offenders," Bureau of Justice Statistics, 1997.

13. Association for the Treatment of Sexual Abusers.

14. The CSOM provides training and support to jurisdictions for sexual offender management. The CSOM is an initiative supported by the U.S. Department of Justice, Office of Justice Programs, the National Institute of Corrections, and the State Justice Institute. The project is administered by the agencies, with the Center for Effective Public Policy and the American Probation and Parole Association.

15. Mike Lew, *Victims No Longer: Men Recovering from Incest and Child Sexual Abuse* (New York: HarperCollins, 1990), p. 243. Lew's thorough Chapter 18, on confrontation, is an excellent resource for women as well as men.

16. Incest and Sexual Abuse Legal Resource Kit, 1995; NOW Legal Defense and Education Fund. The $5 kit is a good general information resource, though it is not meant to be used in place of consultation with a lawyer. The kit can be obtained by writing NOW Legal Defense and Education Fund, 99 Hudson Street, New York, NY 10013, or by ordering online at http://www.nowldef.org/html/pub/form.shtml.

17. Much of this information has been drawn from the National Center for Victims of Crime's "Civil Justice for Victims of Crime" pamphlet, the NOW Legal Defense and Education Fund's Incest and Sexual Abuse Legal Resource Kit, the National Crime Victim Bar Association, and the Rosa Parks Sexual Assault Crisis Center in Los Angeles.

18. Compiled from "Civil Justice for Victims of Crime," the National Crime Victim Bar Association, and the National Center for Victims of Crime.

Chapter Eight: Reconciliation . . . and Moving On

1. Ellen Bass and Laura Davis, *The Courage to Heal: A Guide for Women Survivors of Child Sexual Abuse,* 3rd ed. (New York: Harper Perennial, 1998), p. 151.

2. *Newsweek* poll, November 10, 2003.

3. Marcia L. Dyson, "When Preachers Prey," *Essence*, May 1998, p. 120.

4. http://www.voices-action.org/How%20To%20Confront.htm;   cited April 24, 2003. VOICES stands for Victims of Incest Can Emerge Survivors, an international victims support and public awareness organization. You can request this information in a pamphlet from VOICES in Action, Inc., P.O. Box 148309, Chicago, IL 60614.

BIBLIOGRAPHY

Abney, Veronica D., and Ronnie Priest. "African Americans and Child Sexual Abuse." In Lisa Aronson Fontes, ed., *Sexual Abuse in Nine North American Cultures: Treatment and Prevention.* Thousand Oaks, CA: Sage Publications, 1995.

Ainscough, Carolyn, and Kay Toon. *Breaking Free: A Self-Help Guide for Adults Who Were Sexually Abused as Children.* Tucson: Fisher Books, 1993.

Bass, Ellen, and Laura Davis. *The Courage to Heal: A Guide for Women Survivors of Child Sexual Abuse,* 3rd ed. New York: Harper Perennial, 1994.

Blume, E. Sue. *Secret Survivors: Uncovering Incest and Its Aftereffects in Women.* New York: Ballantine Books, 1990

Boyd-Franklin, Nancy. *Black Families in Therapy: A Multisystems Approach.* New York: The Guilford Press, 1989.

Boyd-Franklin, Nancy, A. J. Franklin, and Pamela Toussaint. *Boys into Men: Raising Our African American Teenage Sons.* New York: Plume, 2000.

Cole, Johnetta Betsch, and Beverly Guy-Sheftall. *Gender Talk: The Struggle for Women's Equality in African American Communities.* New York: Ballantine Books, 2003.

Cooper-White, Pamela. *The Cry of Tamar: Violence Against Women and the Church's Response.* Minneapolis: Fortress Press, 1995.

Crinch, Joseph E., and Kimberly A. Crinch. *Shifting the Burden of Truth: Suing Child Sexual Abusers—A Legal Guide for Survivors and Their Supporters.* Lake Oswego, OR: Recollex Publishing, 1992.

Dugan, Meg Kennedy, and Roger Hock. *It's My Life Now: Starting Over After an Abusive Relationship or Domestic Violence.* New York: Routledge, 2000.

Finkelhor, David. *A Sourcebook on Child Sexual Abuse.* Thousand Oaks, CA: Sage Publications, 1986.

———. *Child Sexual Abuse: New Theory & Research.* New York: The Free Press, 1984.

———. *Sexually Victimized Children.* New York: The Free Press, 1979.

Fout, John C., and Maura Shaw Tantillo, eds. *American Sexual Politics: Sex, Gender and Race Since the Civil War.* Chicago: University of Chicago Press, 1993.

Fox-Genovese, Elizabeth. *Within the Plantation Household: Black and White Women of the Old South.* Chapel Hill: University of North Carolina Press, 1988.

Gaspar, David Barry, and Darlene Clark Hine, eds. *More Than Chattel: Black Women and Slavery in the Americas.* Bloomington: Indiana University Press, 1996.

Lew, Mike. *Victims No Longer: Men Recovering from Incest and Other Sexual Child Abuse.* New York: HarperCollins, 1986.

Matsakis, Aphrodite. *I Can't Get Over It: A Handbook for Trauma Survivors,* 2nd ed. Oakland, CA: New Harbinger Publications, 1996.

Monahon, Cynthia. *Children and Trauma: A Guide for Parents and Professionals.* San Francisco: Jossey-Bass Publishers, 1993.

Newberger, Eli H. *The Men They Will Become: The Nature and Nurture of Male Character.* Cambridge, MA: Perseus Publishing, 1999.

Parham, Thomas A., Joseph L. White, and Adisa Ajamu. *The Psychology of Blacks: An African-Centered Perspective,* 3rd ed. Upper Saddle River, NJ: Prentice Hall, 2000.

Paymar, Michael. *Violent No More: Helping Men End Domestic Abuse.* Alameda, CA: Hunter House, 1993.

Pryor, Douglas W. *Unspeakable Acts: Why Men Sexually Abuse Children.* New York: New York University Press, 1996.

Richardson, Brenda, and Brenda Wade. *What Mama Couldn't Tell Us About Love: Healing the Emotional Legacy of Racism by Celebrating Our Light.* New York: Perennial, 2000.

Robinson, Lori S. *I Will Survive: The African-American Guide to Healing from Sexual Assault and Abuse*. New York: Seal Press, 2002.

Seamands, David A. *Healing for Damaged Emotions*. Colorado Springs: Chariot Victor Books, 1991.

Shapiro, Francine, and Margot Silk Forrest. *EMDR: The Breakthrough "Eye Movement" Therapy for Overcoming Anxiety, Stress, and Trauma*. New York: Basic Books, 1997.

Somé, Malidoma Patrice. *Ritual: Power, Healing, and Community*. New York: Penguin Compass, 1993.

———. *The Healing Wisdom of Africa*. New York: Tarcher/Putnam, 1998.

West, Carolyn M. *Violence in the Lives of Black Women: Battered, Black, and Blue*. New York: Haworth Press, 2002.

West, Traci C. *Wounds of the Spirit*. New York: New York University Press, 1999.

White, Deborah Gray. *Ar'n't I a Woman? Female Slaves in the Plantation South*. New York: W. W. Norton and Co., 1999.

White, Evelyn C. *The Black Women's Health Book. Speaking for Ourselves*. Seattle: Seal Press, 1990.

Wyatt, Gail E. *Stolen Women*. New York: John Wiley & Sons, Inc., 1997.

Wyatt, Gail E., and Gloria Johnson Powell, eds. *Lasting Effects of Child Sexual Abuse*. Thousand Oaks, CA: Sage Publications, 1988.

Wyatt, Gail E., Michael D. Newcomb, and Monika H. Riederle. *Sexual Abuse and Consensual Sex: Women's Developmental Patterns and Outcomes*. Thousand Oaks, CA: Sage Publications, 1993.

INDEX

A

abusers, 9

  accountability, 212–13

  acquaintances, 12, 15, 37–38, 43, 107–8, 126, 158–59

  apology and amends or reparations, 213

  of boys, 152

  characteristics, 121–23, 174

  child pornography and, 175

  confronting, 209–12

  extended family of, 58, 143

  family members, 3, 12, 15, 16, 20, 37, 41–43, 45–46, 52, 53, 56–58, 61–72, 77, 85, 99, 100–101, 103–4, 119, 123–25, 127, 138, 162–67, 185–90, 204–5, 208, 210–11

  help for, 42, 58, 83, 175–77

  Internet predators, 145

  isolation and, 83, 177

  legal action against, 16, 56, 176, 208 (see also reporting; legal action)

  most common, 12, 120

  motivation of, 121, 122

  parents of, 56–58

  pedophilia and adolescence, 167–68, 174

  power and, 12, 122

  preconditions for abuse to occur, 122 23, 173

  Sex Offender Registry, 122

  sexual compulsions and, 173, 177

  spouses/partners of, 56

  stopping, 9 (see also protection of children against abuse)

  strangers, 12, 120

  substance abuse and, 174, 176, 186, 195

  supervision and treatment, 175–77, 195–97, 212

  tricks and tools used by, 125–28

  uncles as, 3, 17, 37, 53, 204, 208, 221, 224

  what makes them tick, 173–75

addiction, alcoholism, or substance abuse, 12, 21, 37, 38, 39, 41, 58, 97–101, 140, 152, 164–65, 220

African Americans

  depression, prevalence of, 80

  effects of abuse and, 53

  facts about sexual abuse and, 53

  faith and prayer, 214, 216

  family, characterizations of, 53–54

  family, importance of, 205

  rape and, 17

  protecting the race, 29

reactions to sexual abuse, 17
reporting abuse, 36
sexual abuse among, 14–16
slavery, legacy of, 26–31, 54, 133,
    163
therapy, attitudes about, 81, 82–83
Ainscough, Carolyn, 38
Ajamu, Adisa, 83
Almeida, Rhea, 83, 132, 197, 198,
    206, 207, 210, 212, 213, 214,
    218
American Art Therapy Association,
    92
American Bar Association, 202
American Music Therapy
    Association, 92
American Psychiatric Association,
    175
American Society of Clinical
    Hypnosis, 93
anxiety, 39, 80, 104
Association of Black Psychologists, 88
Aya Model, 115–18

B

Bass, Ellen, 55
Basso, Michael J., 134
"Behind the Mask" (Dyson), 151
bibliotherapy, 85, 94–95
blame, 123, 143, 181
    boys as victims and, 152–53, 158
    victim and, 25, 136, 141
Blume, E. Sue, 15
body memory, 95–96
Boyd-Franklin, Nancy, 30, 53, 59
boys and men as survivors, 13, 15,
    149–71

abusers of, most common, 152
advice for parents or caregivers,
    169–70
common issues, 167–68
concerns about masculinity and
    homophobia, 151–53
depression and sexual abuse, 12
difficulty verbalizing feelings,
    155–56
effects of sexual abuse, 151–52
"emotional prison" of, 150
encouragement and support for,
    169
females as abusers of, 154–55, 157
homosexuality, confusion about,
    153–55, 164, 165
men helping men, 171
nondisclosure of sexual abuse, 152
pedophilia and adolescence,
    167–68, 174
sexually related problems and
    likeliness to victimize others,
    153, 156
societal costs, 156–57
steps to take for dealing with
    abuse, 170
substance abuse and, 152
supermacho image, 156
women helping men, 171
*Breaking Free: A Self-Help Guide for
    Adults Who Were Sexually Abused
    as Children* (Ainscough and
    Toon), 38, 49

C

Center for Gender Equality, 23
Center for Sex Offender Manage-

ment (Silver Spring, MD), 177, 179

Child Abuse Prevention and Treatment Act (CAPTA), 121

Childhelp USA, 147

Child's Bill of Rights, 148

Church, Pam, 135–37, 158

Coalition on Child Abuse and Neglect, 125

confidence, lack of, 2, 39

Cose, Ellis, 156

counseling, 57
  effective, 6
  finding the right therapist, 87–90
  importance of, 46
  ineffective, 6
  for male survivors, 170
  recommending, 76, 81, 105
  therapeutic themes, common, 47–48, 112–13
  See also healing practices; psychotherapy

counselors, survivors as, 19, 21, 96, 97, 101, 107–12, 114, 125, 144, 157–62

Courage to Heal, The (Bass and Davis), 55, 92, 210, 226
  Workbook, 99

crisis centers and hotlines, 88, 147

culture, African American
  children in, 4
  hip-hop movement, 150–51
  homophobia in, 152, 153
  silence about sexual abuse in, 29
  slavery, legacy of, 26–31, 54, 133, 163
  women in, 4, 29

culture, American
  boys and men, repression of feminine qualities and emotions, 150
  messages that make children targets of abuse, 22–26
  violence in, 8, 25

Cunningham, Dorothy, 46, 47, 127–28, 131, 206

D

Darkness to Light (Charleston, SC), 145, 146

Davis, Janet, 84, 205, 206, 218–19, 229

Davis, Laura, 55

delinquency, 98, 140, 157, 192–93

Department of Child Protective Services, MI, 138

depression, 9, 13, 15, 21, 39, 40, 77–78, 80, 81, 102, 104, 143, 159, 208
  symptoms of, sexual abuse and, 140

disclosure, 5–6, 20, 47–48
  acknowledging and validating child's experience, 138–39, 147, 179, 206
  behavior as, 55
  breaking the silence, 49–51
  confrontation and, 211–12, 226–29
  reasons for, 20, 48, 143–44, 179
  responding, supportive ways, 76, 146–47, 169–71
  response, denial as, 18, 42, 43, 46, 61, 96, 120, 206

responses, common, 52, 61,
    72–74, 96, 143, 159, 206–7
"secondary injuries," 21, 42
ways to start a conversation about
    possible abuse, 75
why children don't tell, 49–51,
    107, 108
dissociation, 27, 34
Dugan, Meg Kennedy, 23–24,
    25–26
Dyson, Marcia, 214, 215–16, 218
Dyson, Michael Eric, 151, 171

E
eating disorders, 39, 41, 45, 142
effects of abuse (psychological, emo-
    tional, and behavioral), 2, 4, 6,
    7, 9, 12, 15–16, 21–22, 27, 37,
    38, 39, 77–78, 79, 182–83, 220
    African Americans, 53
    degree of damage, factors in,
        38–39
    flashbacks, 27, 39, 105–6, 159,
        161, 221
    four major ways abuse causes
        problems for survivors, 35
    most common (listing), 39
Emberley, Michael, 134
Essence magazine, 1, 134, 207
eye movement desensitization and
    reprocessing (EMDR), 92–93

F
family, 52–53
    abuse in, effects, 7, 9, 55–58,
        178–95
    abuse as open secret in, 60–72

    African American, 53–54
    African American "umbrella of"
        or extended, 20, 30, 58
    common responses to disclosure
        of abuse, 73–74, 139, 141–43
    denial, 18, 43, 46
    dynamics or dysfunction and sex-
        uality, 43, 53, 54–55, 60–72,
        84, 141, 143, 162–67
    fear of disrupting or losing
        through disclosure, 204–6
    "one for all" attitude, 30, 164
    parents of abusers, 56–58
    renegotiating relationship with,
        205–6
    responsibilities of, 17–19
    rules, unspoken, 4–5
    secrets, 59, 134, 141
    siblings of survivors, 55–56, 183
    silence, 4, 7, 40, 43
    spouses/partners of abusers, 56
    substance abuse in, and sexual
        abuse, 37, 141
    therapy for, 42, 84
Family Code of Conduct, 229–30
fears, 97–98, 104
    of abuser, 49–50, 191
    of disrupting or losing family
        through disclosure, 204–6
    facing, 35
    four major ways abuse causes, 35
    of impending doom, 27
    terror or fear of lack of safety, 15,
        102–3
    why children don't tell and, 49–50
Finkelhor, David, 35, 122–23
Fisher, Antwone, 155

flashbacks, 27, 39, 105–6, 159,
    161, 221
Ford, Bill, 173, 176, 195

G
Good Touch/Bad Touch® curricu-
    lum, 135–37, 148
Grant, Gwendolyn Goldsby, 134
Green, Chimene, 94

H
Harris, Robie, 134
Hartsfield, Jeanne, 194
healers, 96–97
healing
    accountability, 212–13
    acknowledgment, 95–96
    action, 96–97
    apology and/or amends and repa-
        rations, 206, 212, 213
    coming to terms with abusers,
        218–19
    confrontation, 209–12, 226–29
    faith and forgiveness, 213–18
    finding resolution, 207–8
    journaling, 185, 204, 208,
        219–23
    legal action and, 201, 208
    letter of loss, 227–29
    letting go/letting God, 223–25
    lonely journey to, 142–44
    male survivors, steps to take for
        dealing with abuse, 170
    reconciliation and moving on,
        204–25
    renegotiating relationship with
        family, 205–6

severing family ties, 205
stages of progress, 95–97, 105–7
understanding, 96
validation and, 206
healing practices, 9, 47–48
    Aya Model, 115–18
    bibliotherapy, 85, 94–95
    cognitive therapy, 82
    couples therapy, 84–87
    creative (art, music, dance, writ-
        ing), 47, 91–92, 210, 211, 212
    eye movement desensitization
        and reprocessing (EMDR),
        92–93
    family therapy, 84, 182
    finding the right therapist, 87–90
    health insurance, 88
    hypnotherapy, 93
    massage or bodywork, 93–94
    mental health centers, 208, 219
    referrals, 88
    Reiki, 94, 214
    talk therapy (group), 83, 192
    talk therapy (individual psy-
        chotherapy), 47, 66, 78–80,
        81–83, 105–6, 166, 182, 192
health problems and sexual abuse,
    14, 15, 37, 40, 46
Hicks, Ronda, 125
Hill, Anita, 29
HIV risk, 15, 16, 153
Hock, Roger, 23–24, 25–26
homosexuality
    confusion about sexual identity
        and, 153–55, 164, 165
    homophobia in African American
        community, 152, 153

I

Institute for Family Services
(Somerset, NJ), 83, 132, 197,
210, 212
International Association of Reiki
Professionals, 94
Internet
American Bar Association, 202
American Society of Clinical
Hypnosis, 93
Darkness to Light, 145
Good Touch/Bad Touch®, 148
Justice for Children, 202
Martindale-Hubbell Lawyer
Locator, 202
National Bar Association, 202
National Center for Victims of
Crime, 203
National Crime Victim Bar
Association, 202
National Organization for Victim
Assistance (NOVA), 199
predators on, 145
Rape, Abuse & Incest National
Network (RAINN), 203
Susan Smith, attorney at law, 203
*It's So Amazing! A Book About Eggs,
Sperm, Birth, Babies, and Families*
(Harris and Emberley), 134

J

Justice for Children, 147, 194, 202

K

Kanka, Megan, 121–22
King, Eileen, 194–95

L

legal action, 16, 56, 177, 197–201
civil suit, 199–201
convictions of sex offenders, 175
criminal prosecution, 199
difficulties of pressing charges,
197–98, 199
finding a lawyer, 202
flaws in the system, 194–95
incarceration and parole, 175–77,
194
percentage of cases prosecuted,
172
preparing for the attorney, 202–3
questions to consider before pursuing, 198
resolving history and healing,
201, 208
sex offenders, fast facts about,
176
statutes of limitations, 203
Lew, Mike, 154, 166
Lewis, Diane, 34
Little Mermaid, The (film), 132

M

Martindale-Hubbell Lawyer
Locator, 202
massage or bodywork, 93–94
Matson, Scott, 177, 179
medication, 105, 107
Megan's Law, 121–22
Morrison, Toni, 29
Murray, Carmen, 138–40, 214, 217
Mustardseed (Brooklyn, NY), 173,
176, 195–97

N

Narcotics Anonymous, 98
National Bar Association, 202
National Center for Victims of
    Crime, 203
National Child Abuse Hotline, 147
National Crime Victim Bar Associ-
    ation, 202
National Organization for Victim
    Assistance (NOVA), 199
Newberger, Eli, 155–56
Northside Center for Children,
    New York City, 84, 205

P

PAM Programs, 148
Parham, Thomas A., 83
perfectionism, 4, 37, 79, 107
powerlessness, 5, 35
Project Greenhope, Manhattan,
    NY (alternative to incarcera-
    tion), 44
prostitution, 16, 38, 43–44
protection of children against abuse,
    9, 30
    community notification pro-
        grams, 175
    four preconditions for abuse to
        occur, 122–23, 173
    identifying sexualized children,
        138–39
    information about sex, 120, 130
    listening to children, 131, 146–47
    raising thinking children, 132–33
    recognizing sexuality, 133–35
    risk factors, 128–29, 181
    seven steps for, 145–46

    sexual versus sexualized children,
        137–38
    signs of distress, 139–40
    talking about good touch/bad
        touch, 135–37
Pryor, Douglas, 126
Psychology of Blacks, The (Parham,
    White, and Ajamu), 83, 114–15
psychotherapy
    for abusers, 176–77
    African-centered, 114–15
    cognitive therapy, 82
    couples therapy, 84–87, 107,
        109–12
    family therapy, 84, 182
    talk therapy (group), 83, 192
    talk therapy (individual psycho-
        therapy), 47, 66, 78–80, 81–83,
        99–100, 105–6, 166, 182, 192
PTSD (post-traumatic stress
    disorder), 32

R

Rape, Abuse & Incest National
    Network (RAINN), 88, 203
Reiki, 94
relationships
    couples therapy, 84–87, 107,
        109–12
    problems of survivors, 39, 41–42,
        99, 143, 159, 165, 221, 222
    spouses/partners of abusers, 46
    spouses/partners of survivors,
        84–87, 159
reporting sexual abuse, 16–17, 36,
    147, 169, 172–73, 177, 194
    boys and reluctance, 152, 153

mandatory, 121
statistics, 120
See also legal action
resolution
accountability, 212–13
confrontation, 209–12, 226–29
faith and forgiveness, 213–18
finding, 207–8
responses to abuse
dismissing, 35, 42, 155
minimizing, 35, 96, 155
pleasure/repulsion dichotomy,
46–47, 127
rationalizing, 35, 155
self-blame, 35
See also effects of abuse
Richardson, Brenda, 22–23, 26–27,
38
Rosa Parks Sexual Assault Crisis
Center, Los Angeles, CA, 194

S

secrets
abuse as open, 59–72
common within families, 59
deception, 59
open, 59, 108–9
rape, 107
self-esteem
giving children a voice and, 135
lowered, 9, 152
strong, and ability to think critically, 132–33
self-mutilation, 21, 102, 140, 220
"7 Steps to Protecting Children
from Sexual Abuse," 145–46
Sex Offender Registry, 122

sexual abuse
age of greatest vulnerability, 120
boys and, 13, 15, 149–71 (*see also*
boys and men as survivors)
coping strategies (hidden signs of
abuse), 141–42
degree of damage, factors in,
38–39
four preconditions for abuse to
occur, 122–23, 173
girls and, 13, 15
how big is the problem, 14–16
how children are easy prey,
123–24
incest, 12, 53, 140–41
power and, 12–13
range of, 12, 53
risk factors, 128–30, 181
signs of, 139–40
societal costs, 16, 156–57
victims, highest risk category, 120
"what happened?" questions to ask
yourself, 13–14
what it is, 8, 154
sexual information and education,
120, 130, 137–38
books recommended, 134
Good Touch/Bad Touch® curriculum, 135–37
recognizing children's sexuality,
133–35
sexual language, 25–26
sexual promiscuity or risky behavior, 6, 15–16, 38, 98, 109, 120,
140, 165, 192, 204, 220
shame and guilt, 5, 36–39, 40, 123,
141, 216

Shange, Ntozake, 29
signs of abuse, 55, 139–40
    coping strategies (hidden signs
        of abuse), 141–42
    questions to ask, 32–33
sleep disorders, 27, 140
"sleepwalking," 34
Sloan, Victoria J., 155, 156
Smith, Susan, attorney at law, 203
Somé, Malidoma, 115, 116
stigmatization, 35
Stop It Now (Haydenville, MA),
    175
suicide, 21, 37, 38, 39, 48, 81, 102,
    105, 140, 182, 208, 222
support systems, 42, 44–45, 57, 80,
    81, 184
    for male survivors, 170
survivors, 8–9
    blaming the victim, 25, 138
    boys and men as survivors, 13,
        15, 149–71
    characteristics of targets, 22–26
    most common categories, 12–13
    victim-survivors, 13
    "what happened?" questions to ask
        yourself, 13–14
    See also effects of abuse; healing
symptoms. See signs of abuse

T
Taylor, Susan, 1, 6
therapy. See psychotherapy; healing
    practices
Thomas, Clarence, 29
Toon, Kay, 38
traumatic sexualization, 35

Truth and Reconciliation Commis-
    sion, South Africa, 213
Turner, Maelinda, 32, 34, 40, 41,
    42, 47, 82, 88, 90, 92, 206,
    214, 216–17
Tyson, Mike, 29

U
Underground Guide to Teenage Sexual-
    ity, The (Basso), 134
Unspeakable Acts: Why Men Sexually
    Abuse Children (Pryor), 126

V
Victims No Longer: Men Recovering
    from Incest and Other Sexual Abuse
    (Lew), 154, 166
VOICES (Victims of Incest Can
    Emerge Survivors), 88
VOICES in Action, Inc., 226

W
Wade, Brenda, 26–27
Walker, Alice, 29
Wallace, Michele, 29
Washington, Desiree, 29
Wattleton, Faye, 23, 24
Wells-Wilbon, Rhonda, 114–15
    Aya Model, 115–18
West, Traci, 13, 25, 36, 47
White, Joseph L., 83
withdrawal, 4, 39, 103, 140
women
    African American, myths, 28–31
    cultural messages that make them
        targets for abuse, 22–25
    depression and, 80, 81

socialization, countering negative,
    132–33
violence against, 4, 8, 25–26,
    37
worthlessness, feelings of, 45, 53

Wyatt, Gail E., 15, 17, 18, 27,
    43, 44

Y
YWCA, 88

ROBIN D. STONE is a former Executive Editor of *Essence* magazine and the founding Editor-in-Chief of essence.com. She was also an editor for the *New York Times,* the *Boston Globe,* the *Detroit Free Press,* and *Family Circle,* and has written for numerous publications, including *Essence* and *Glamour.* She was a Kaiser Media Fellow in 2002–2003, and she teaches journalism at New York University. A Detroit native, she lives in New York City with her husband and their son.

Made in the USA
Middletown, DE
24 February 2021

34332234R00182